EXERCISE EVERY DAY

32 TACTICS FOR BUILDING THE EXERCISE HABIT

(EVEN IF YOU HATE WORKING OUT)

BY: S.J. SCOTT

www.HabitBooks.com

ISBN: 1511767057
ISBN-13: 978-1511767057

Disclaimer

No part of this publication may be reproduced or transmitted in any form or by any means, mechanical or electronic, including photocopying or recording, or by any information storage and retrieval system, or transmitted by email without permission in writing from the publisher.

While all attempts have been made to verify the information provided in this publication, neither the author nor the publisher assumes any responsibility for errors, omissions, or contrary interpretations of the subject matter herein.

This book is for entertainment purposes only. The views expressed are those of the author alone, and should not be taken as expert instruction or commands. The reader is responsible for his or her own actions.

Adherence to all applicable laws and regulations, including international, federal, state, and local laws governing professional licensing, business practices, advertising, and all other aspects of doing business in the US, Canada, or any other jurisdiction is the sole responsibility of the purchaser or reader.

Neither the author nor the publisher assumes any responsibility or liability whatsoever on the behalf of the purchaser or reader of these materials.

Any perceived slight of any individual or organization is purely unintentional.

YOUR FREE GIFT

As a way of saying *thanks* for your purchase, I'm offering a free report that's exclusive to my book and blog readers.

In *77 Good Habits to Live a Better Life*, you'll discover a variety of routines that can help you in many different areas of your life. You will learn how to make lasting changes to your work, success, learning, health, and sleep habits.

Go Here to Grab 77 Good Habits to Live a Better Life:

www.developgoodhabits.com/free

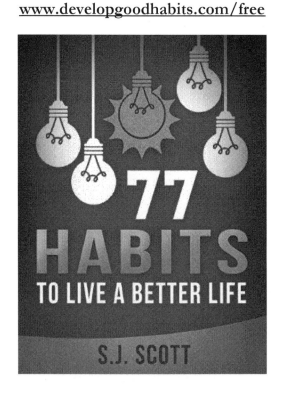

Table of Contents

INTRODUCTION

How to Exercise Every Day

Wish you had time to exercise? Are you turned off by the "meat-market" scene at most gyms, or are you simply unsure about how to get started?

You aren't alone.

The good news is that you don't have to follow extreme exercise programs like Insanity and P90X, or spend every free moment in the gym to experience the health benefits exercise has to offer. All you need to do is make a simple goal to "Exercise Every Day" in a way that fits your already busy schedule.

Here's the thing—most people have both the desire and capacity to exercise, but they never get started because they allow obstacles to get in their way.

For instance, you might feel exhausted when your alarm clock goes off two hours earlier than usual in the morning, so you can't bring yourself to make it to "boot camp" class.

Or perhaps you don't have space in your house for lots of weights and equipment.

These are real-life obstacles, and it's likely that issues such as these have prevented you from engaging in regular exercise.

In this book, **Exercise Every Day**, you will have the opportunity to identify those obstacles that seem to continually get in your way.

Then you will learn how to review each obstacle and identify the specific solutions you can use to experience a personal breakthrough

Finally, while many books on exercise provide a generalized list of tips, I take things a step further by helping you learn why a specific strategy works, what limiting belief it eliminates, and how you can immediately apply the strategy to your life.

Who Am I?

My name is Steve "S.J." Scott. I run the blog Develop Good Habits, and I'm the author of a series of habit-related titles, all of which are available at **HabitBooks.com**.

The purpose of my content is to show how continuous habit development can lead to a better life. Instead of lecturing you, I provide simple strategies that are easy to use no matter how busy you get during the day.

While I'm not a personal trainer, I do consider myself to be someone who has **successfully built the exercise habit over the last 25 years**.

My credentials: I've completed fifteen marathons. In the last year or so, I've developed the habit of walking an average of 10,000 steps per day. I also enjoy a multitude of other activities such as biking, surfing, and swimming. Finally, I often combine traveling with achieving major athletic goals—including a recent trip to Tanzania to hike up Mount Kilimanjaro.

The common thread of all these accomplishments is that I've maintained the exercise habit throughout my life—no matter what obstacle popped up along the way. In fact, it's because of these obstacles that I've been able to create simple but effective strategies to consistently exercise on a daily basis. I detail many of these strategies in this book.

About Exercise Every Day

The purpose of this book isn't to lecture you or make you feel bad. Rather, **Exercise Every Day** is designed to help you clear up a few common misconceptions about exercise, identify your personal obstacles, and implement real-life solutions for developing a lifelong exercise habit.

I've found—by talking to people from all walks of life—that most of us have a skewed viewpoint of exercise.

On one end of the spectrum are "exercise gurus" who make you believe that exercise is only effective if you do something like P90X, Insanity, running marathons, or spending two hours in the gym. On the other end of the spectrum, there are those who barely move during the day.

Exercise doesn't have to be a black-and-white, all-or-nothing proposition.

The better solution is to create a sustainable habit, enabling you to get the right amount of exercise for your unique situation. Before creating this new habit, it's important to understand why you have failed to build an exercise routine in the past and how you can take practical steps to overcome these challenges.

The truth is that people who exercise regularly don't have more motivation than others. They feel tired, uncomfortable, and busy just like everyone else. The difference that spurs them into action is having an established habit that pushes them beyond excuses.

Exercise Every Day doesn't focus on any one particular type of exercise. It is designed to help you build any type of exercise habit, from weight lifting to yoga, CrossFit to sports, or swimming to walking.

For this reason, **Exercise Every Day** doesn't cover specific details for each type of exercise. Instead, I focus on how to develop the proper mindset, which will allow you to build the right habits for your personal success. Then I'll provide a simple action plan for getting started with an exercise routine that fits your personal situation.

This book has a straightforward layout. Each section starts with a major obstacle that people encounter when building the exercise habit. Then, for each obstacle, I provide a few actionable strategies you can use to overcome it. In total, there are 32 real-life solutions to these common challenges. By the time you're done, you'll understand the "why" behind your personal obstacles and "how" you can overcome them.

There is wealth of material to cover, so let's start by talking about obstacles and how they often prevent people from exercising on a consistent basis.

The Truth About Exercise Obstacles

This book started with a simple email.

A few months back, I emailed my list of subscribers and asked them about the one habit they would most like to build. After reading more than 400 responses, I realized that many people struggle with their health and fitness.

The interesting thing?

Most already knew what they had to do, but they didn't know how to overcome the obstacles they often faced. In fact, many felt it was because of these challenges that they weren't able to exercise on a regular basis.

The truth is, a lack of desire isn't what prevents most people from exercising. Instead, people tend to allow obstacles to derail their efforts. That means the trick to building the exercise habit is to know how to do it regularly—even when you continually experience those pesky challenges.

To illustrate this point, let me briefly (and hopefully humorously) describe the various obstacles I've encountered in my 25 years of a running. In fact, there have been so many "incidents" that I have to categorize them.

VARIOUS INJURIES

Pericarditis. Shin splints. Torn hamstring. Heat exhaustion. Plantar fasciitis. Dancer's hip. (Seriously, I have something called dancer's hip. Look it up, it's a real thing.)

ANIMAL ATTACKS

Chased by a fast three-legged dog. (Okay, this wasn't that scary, but it was one of the odder moments of my life.) Sideswiped by a 12-point buck during a college cross-country race. Bitten (and chased up a hill) by a farm dog while running through the French countryside. Pursued by a pack of seven dachshunds. (Again, not too scary, but those little guys sure can bite.)

PEOPLE

Cars swerving at me. Having random objects thrown at me: glass bottles, rocks, even a piece of pizza. Had a driver get out of a car and chase me five blocks through Newark, New Jersey. And my personal favorite: hearing "Run, Forrest, run!" for the past 20 years.

BAD WEATHER

There have been countless days when I've had to deal with scorching heat, torrential rain, and icy roads.

BRUCE SPRINGSTEEN

Seriously, one day, Bruce Springsteen almost ran me over when he pulled out of his driveway. Yes, that Bruce Springsteen.

Okay, I'll admit that some of these obstacles could have been avoided with better planning on my part.

My point in talking about them here is to show that when you do an activity on a regular basis, you're bound to encounter a few obstacles along the way. The trick is to learn how to not only respond to them, but also prevent many of them from happening in the first place.

And that's what we'll cover throughout this book!

Based on those 400 email responses, I've uncovered **seven common obstacles** to building the exercise habit and developed a total of 32 real-life solutions to help you tackle them head-on. There is a lot to cover, so let's get to it.

OBSTACLE (1):

LACK OF KNOWLEDGE

I f you are new to exercising, chances are these are some of the questions that go through your mind:

- *What weights do I use?*
- *How do I get started?*
- *When do I stretch?*
- *What exercise is appropriate for my age?*
- *What do I need to do to drop 20 pounds/get fitter/look awesome in my swimsuit/get healthy/_____ (fill in the blank for your personal goal)?*

I am big on goals and plans. I understand the need to have some answers and have direction, but the problem is that some people want to have all the answers before they start. This indecision can often prevent you from starting an exercise program, so the best thing you can do is stop researching and just start moving.

> *"Knowing is half the battle."*
> — G.I. Joe

Does this quote speak to you?

Do you find that lack of knowledge holds you back?

There's a term for the phenomenon of needing to ask questions and have all of the information you need before getting started. It's called "paralysis by analysis."

This phenomenon happens when you have too much information coming at you from too many different directions, especially when one piece of information contradicts another.

Instead of deciding to move forward and take action, you feel frozen. In essence, you're paralyzed by too many pieces of information. You do nothing and walk away from it all feeling frustrated and confused. (Here's a great article that further explains the dangers of information overload:

http://bit.ly/1ChDbbR)

In this section, we'll talk about how to find the right exercise program (for you) and then cover a few tactics for getting started. Obviously, the trick is to take action. Only YOU will know what exercises are right for you, so let this be the day you let go of "analysis paralysis" and move forward with your new goal.

Tactic #1: Start at the End

In order to exercise on a regular basis, you need a clear picture of your long-term goals. This means identifying what you most want in life and then working your way backward.

As an example, do any of the following goals sound familiar?

- Get ripped?
- Look sexy?
- Lose weight?
- Be healthier?

Think carefully about what you want from an exercise routine. It will help determine the right program for you. In other words, an older woman who wants to improve her overall health will probably follow a much different routine from the guy who wants that ripped look.

Next, identify how much time you honestly have to devote to exercising.

Less than 30 minutes? 30 to 60 minutes? 60+ minutes every day?

Be honest with yourself here. If your time is already limited, then don't expect to adhere to a strict *P90X* program that requires a two-hour daily commitment. Instead, look for something that fits into your hectic schedule.

HOW TO IMPLEMENT

Step One:

To get started, you must...*identify your desires*!

Ask yourself the questions we discussed before to narrow down your specific goals.

Do you want to:

- Get ripped?
- Look sexy?
- Lose weight?
- Be healthier?

Yes, some types of exercise will produce multiple positive results. However, you need to identify the specific results you want so you can pick the right routine.

Step Two:

Ask additional questions that help narrow down your personal goals. For example:

- Is increasing stamina, flexibility, or muscle growth more important to you?
- Do you prefer exercising inside or outside?
- Do want to do high-impact or low-impact exercises?
- Do you want to work out alone or with a group?
- Do you prefer to go to a gym or to work out at home?
- Do you have any physical limitations that might prevent you from doing certain types of exercise?

Be honest with these answers. They are the key to identifying the right program for your hectic schedule.

Step Three:

Check out the exercises listed below. You can start with just one exercise or mix and match activities to work toward achieving your goals.

Cardiovascular: Cardiovascular exercise is activity that elevates your heart rate and improves your body's ability to move oxygen through your blood vessels. This type of exercise improves your stamina, breathing, and lung capacity.

Example exercises: running and walking

Strength/resistance training: Strength or resistance training involves using any type of resistance to increase the muscle mass in a certain part of the body. This type of exercise is not just for bodybuilders. Strength training helps improve your posture, your stamina, and the health of your bones. It also helps build lean muscle, which can help you burn more fat.

Example exercises: weight lifting and CrossFit

Flexibility training: Flexibility training helps improve the range of motion in your tendons and joints, making it easier for you to move naturally and fluidly. The primary types of flexibility training are stretching exercises and yoga.

Example exercise: foam rolling and stretching

Balance training: Balance exercises improve your coordination and your agility. These exercises are especially important for older adults because better balance helps to prevent falls.

Example exercise: lunge to balance or step up to balance

Step Four:

You should also consider your interests and preferences when choosing workouts. For example:

- *Don't like the gym?* Create a home-based workout routine.
- *Love the great outdoors?* Consider hiking or find local walking trails.
- *Looking for a workout that calms your mind?* Try yoga!
- *Want to meet new people?* Go to an exercise class.

Finding a workout regimen that matches your goals and preferences may take a little bit of time, but it *is* worth the effort.

If your exercise plan fills you with dread, then it's <u>not</u> the right one for you. In other words, if you absolutely hate doing an activity, it will be hard to keep doing it on a daily basis. However, if your workout plan is interesting and connects with things that you enjoy, then you are much more likely to do it regularly.

Tactic #2: Get Educated

There are probably hundreds (if not thousands) of books discussing specific requirements for all sorts of exercise. Whether you're interested in stretching, running, yoga, weightlifting, or a walking program, you can get details on each with a little bit of research.

Each type of exercise has its own unique features, advantages, and challenges. Once you've picked an exercise program, find two to three resources to learn from. This should help you address any "lack of knowledge" regarding a particular form of exercise. With these resources, you can put yourself ahead of most practitioners in terms of knowledge.

Also, I'd suggest talking to your doctor to see what he or she recommends for your age and level of physical capability. Later on, we'll talk about specific questions you can ask your doctor.

Finally, many exercises require proper technique. One idea is to join a gym and take advantage of the one free personal training session offered to new members. Ask for a customized program and a demonstration for each type of exercise. (We'll talk more about gyms in a later section.)

HOW TO IMPLEMENT

Step One:

Once you have identified a good exercise program, go into research mode. Use resources like YouTube to learn more about proper form for exercises, go to Amazon.com or the library to find books on this subject, listen to podcasts for education from the experts, or use a site like Udemy.com to learn specific, advanced skills.

Step Two:

Listen to (or read/watch) a few resources, taking notes and writing down any questions you may have. You can then take those questions and use Google or another search engine to find your answers.

Step Three:

Resist the urge to keep reading and researching. Remember that "paralysis by analysis" often prevents people from changing their lives. It's easy to get stuck in research mode, so make the decision to cover two to three resources and then commit to taking action.

Tactic #3: Try One Exercise at a Time

So what's another way to overcome paralysis by analysis?

Focus on one exercise at a time.

You may have identified a few different exercise categories that pique your interest, but it is best to start with one and only one. Starting small will help you stay consistent and prevent those feelings of overwhelm.

Do not try to build a "new you" overnight. Putting that kind of pressure on yourself typically leads to failure. This is related to a concept known as ego depletion, which says your ability to focus and resist temptation is reduced throughout the day.

Ego depletion happens when you must constantly use your willpower for certain tasks. The more you use this willpower, the weaker it becomes. If you focus on one task that requires your willpower, you are more likely to accomplish that task. If you spread your willpower out among several tasks, you will likely have a diminished capacity to succeed.

Remember, the goal is not to have a "new you" in one day. That is humanly impossible, anyway. Focus on one thing at a time and build on small wins. A successful exercise habit that will last you a lifetime is built brick by brick by brick.

HOW TO IMPLEMENT

Step One:

Go for the small wins. Pick one exercise to be your focus for the next month. Assign importance to doing this exercise *every day*, even if it is just a quick 15-minute walk. No excuses. Don't let it become one of those things that are continually pushed aside as "more important" things get in the way.

Remember: Distractions will <u>always</u> happen, but you must treat this task as your job to accomplish, no matter what. When you accomplish the task each day, celebrate it as a small win.

Step Two:

Work this task into your daily life. Don't try to make this some major, transformational exercise routine. It should be simple and easy enough to become part of your lifestyle. You don't want this exercise practice to drastically alter your day-to-day schedule. Keep it simple, but make it difficult enough to challenge you.

Step Three:

Make a 30-day commitment to this new exercise routine. Many studies have shown that 30 days is a good length of time for developing a new habit.

It's always hard to get through those first few weeks of a habit change, so this commitment will help you solidify the habit as a new daily behavior. Once you get past this critical 30-day period, it becomes much easier to stick to the routine.

Whether it is walking for fifteen minutes, going to yoga class, or playing basketball with your son, commit to the exercise every day for the next month.

OBSTACLE (2):
LACK OF MOTIVATION

Ever say any of the following to yourself:

- *"I'm tired."*
- *"I just don't feel like it today."*
- *"I just really wish I had some motivation to do it."*
- *"Maybe tomorrow I'll feel more motivated…"*

Sounds familiar, right?

Here's the thing: It's common to feel unmotivated. Most of us have days like this. In fact, most of the people who regularly exercise often feel a lack of motivation before getting started. Yet they take action *despite* these lackluster feelings.

The truth is most people think motivation is required on a daily basis. When they don't feel inspired, they often take a day off. My advice: Never let motivation become the determining factor for getting exercise.

The rah-rah, pithy motivational stuff *doesn't* work. All the cute slogans in the world (like: "beast mode," "just do it," or "push play") won't force you into action. The deciding factor is if you've successfully turned exercise into a regular habit.

Many people beat themselves up because they don't exercise. They often use phrases like "not having willpower," "I'm too lazy," or "I can't do it." What they *don't* realize is willpower is a finite thing. You really can't gut your way through doing a workout.

Oprah Winfrey is a perfect example of this concept.

She is an extremely successful businesswoman and celebrity. It takes an incredible amount of willpower to accomplish what she has accomplished in her lifetime. However, she frequently experiences challenges with her weight. This shows that willpower alone is not enough to stay consistent with any type of habit.

The lesson here is that failure doesn't mean you're "bad" or unsuccessful. When you reach the end of your willpower, you simply don't have the resources to stick to a new habit.

It's been my experience that willpower is like any other muscle. It can be exercised and strengthened over time. The key is to have a structure in place to keep you on track, even when your willpower fails you, and then you can muster the motivation you need.

When it comes to creating the exercise habit, there are many ways to overcome that lack of motivation. In fact, the following solutions will completely take motivation out of the equation.

When you know how to set up your daily schedule, you'll consistently exercise—even on those days when you're not feeling up to it.

Tactic #4: Use "Habit Anchoring"

"Habit anchoring" is a concept that's gained popularity because of B.J. Fogg and his <u>Tiny Habits</u> course. What he recommends is to commit to a very small habit change and then take baby steps as you build upon it. The trick here is to attach the new habit to something you already do on a daily basis.

The example Fogg gives is to create a habit using this recipe:

"After I [your anchor], I will [new habit]."

After you identify the new habit to which you want to commit, identify a routine that you perform on a daily basis. Then attach the new habit to this behavior.

Here are a few examples:

- *"After I sit at my desk in the morning, I will write down my top three priorities for the day."*
- *"After I walk into my home, I will put my keys and wallet/purse on my nightstand."*
- *"After I stop work for the day, I will mentally review the one lesson I learned during my work session."*

Now that you understand what habit anchoring is, let's take a look at the steps you can take to use this technique to achieve your daily exercise goal.

HOW TO IMPLEMENT

Step One:

Identify an automatic habit that you already do without thinking, such as walking to your dresser in the morning, going to your car after work or driving by the gym on your way home. It needs to be something you do nearly every day. If you come up with several routines, think specifically about the ones that take place around the time you'd like to exercise.

Step Two:

Identify the time of day you'd like to exercise, then choose an anchoring habit and schedule a time to get started. Whether this means setting an alarm on your phone, writing it down on a calendar or using a habit-reminder app, the important thing is to pick a time of day when you're mostly likely to succeed. In other words, this will become an appointment you can't and will never break.

Step Three:

Create your habit anchoring statement by filling in the blanks: "After I _____, I will _____."
For instance, you could start with simple statements like these:

- *"After I get into my car after work, I will drive to the gym."*
- *"After I complete my work in the morning, I will take a 10-minute walk before eating lunch."*
- *"After I complete my morning routine, I will complete a five-minute yoga session."*

Get specific with your statement, physically write it on paper, and put it someplace where you can see it. Tape it next to the calendar or on your laptop cover—whatever you have to do to keep this statement in the forefront of your mind.

Finally, you probably noticed that each of these habit anchors has a small goal. That's because it's easier to do something when it's a *micro-commitment*. Let's go over that principle next.

Tactic #5: Make Micro-Commitments

Another reason people lack exercise motivation is that they create goals that are impossible to achieve. They start new exercise routines with huge expectations and a 25-part plan for how they'll experience massive changes. These people often start out strong, but somewhere along the line, their perfect plans fall to pieces.

We've covered some of the primary obstacles and challenges that can throw an exercise routine off its tracks. The problem, however, may not lie with anything that "happens."

The problem could simply be that you are starting with an overly ambitious and rigorous exercise plan. A far better solution is to keep your initial exercise goals simple. Remember, you are developing "exercise every day" habits not "exercise champion" habits.

Making <u>large</u> commitments often becomes *de*-motivational. This is where the hot-cold empathy gap (or HCEG) comes into play. To put it simply, the HCEG is a lack of understanding of the level of temptation you'll feel when encountering a trigger to engage in a bad habit. This trips up many, many people with good intentions.

Consider this: Every New Year, people resolve to change their lives in massive ways. They will drop 20 pounds, cut out major food groups, get buff, eliminate debt, and transform all their interpersonal relationships. In other words, most people make a promise to reinvent themselves during the next 12 months.

The problem with this is that it's hard to remain at that high level of commitment on a daily basis—especially when you have a bad day or experience a major temptation. That initial resolve disappears when people don't account for the rough patches that frequently occur. Most people focus only on their resolutions, not the potential for temptation.

In addition to being prepared for rough patches and temptation, realize that it's more important to keep the streak of daily exercise than it is to do the exercise for a certain length of time, especially when you are building a daily exercise habit.

If you don't have 30 minutes to give to your workout because you had to work late at the office, don't just say, *"Oh, I give up—I don't have time for a full workout."* Instead, work out for 10 or 15 minutes.

My point here is to help you let go of the black-and-white, all-or-nothing thinking. This is about establishing the daily exercise habit, not hitting a specific metric on a daily basis. It's better to be consistent and exercise on a regular basis than it is to have one great workout and then take two days off.

HOW TO IMPLEMENT

Step One:

Make small micro-commitments that make it easy to start the habit. Instead of saying, "I want to drop 20 pounds," say, "I will exercise 20 minutes per day for 30 days." In fact, starting out with a commitment to getting 5 or 10 minutes of exercise daily is enough to develop your habit muscle.

Keep your commitments small and manageable. The idea here is to make the habit so easy that it would seem silly if you didn't do it on a regular basis.

Remember the anchoring statements we discussed? This is a great time to use those as you make your micro-commitments.

For example:

- *"After I get the mail from the mailbox, I will walk around the block."*
- *"After I leave the office, I will stop by the gym to lift weights for 15 minutes."*
- *"After I get the kids to bed, I will practice my stretching for 10 minutes while I watch my favorite show."*

See how that works?

We are talking about small, tiny, micro-commitments.

This is where you begin to add the exercise habit into your life until it becomes second nature, which works especially well for people who think they don't enjoy exercise.

Step Two:

Be prepared for obstacles and temptation. Don't be surprised when you have a bad day or something gets in the way of your micro-commitment.

Stay committed, maintain your focus, and have backup plans in place. Don't accept the excuses your brain will try to come up with. This is a no-excuses plan! For example, if you don't have enough time to exercise in the morning, plan to do your micro-commitment in the evening before bed.

Step Three:

Even if you feel tempted to go bigger with your goal, keep it small, especially in the first 30 days. The goal is to keep your task so small that you cannot fail to achieve it. You need to develop this micro-commitment as a habit before you try to increase your exercise time or go for a bigger goal. The micro-commitment is not a lifetime solution. Once your body adjusts, you can begin to increase difficulty and go for longer exercise times.

To illustrate this point, let's talk about what it's like (for me) to prepare for a marathon. A major component of my training program is running 20 to 22 miles a few times in the final months before an event. Honestly, on many days, the idea of running this distance sounds like a horrific, painful experience. My mental trick is to commit to a goal of 12 to 14 miles; anything "extra" would be unexpected. As weird as it sounds, I give myself "permission" to walk the last few miles if necessary. When I finally get down to those last few miles, I find myself energetic enough to complete all 20 miles of the run.

My point here? It's simple—large commitments can often *prevent* you from exercising because they are so daunting. It's usually hard to get yourself to take action if you think an activity is going to be a grueling experience. It's better to be happy with a smaller outcome, knowing you'll probably do more once you get started.

Step Four:

This section barely scratches the surface of the importance of micro-commitments. In fact, there are three resources on this subject I recommend you check out:

- Mini Habits: Smaller Habits, Bigger Results by Stephen Guise
- Tiny Habits by B.J. Fogg
- Small Move, Big Change: Using Microresolutions to Transform Your Life Permanently by Caroline L. Arnold

Tactic #6: Remove Exercise Obstacles

One way to demotivate yourself is to succumb to the obstacle of not having the "right equipment" to exercise. As an example, let's say you miss a day or two at the gym every month because you forgot to pack a bag of clothes.

The solution?

Be like a Boy Scout and *"always be prepared."*

It's important to have the right exercise equipment on hand, whether you are going to a local gym, exercising in a park, or just planning to work out in your home. My advice is to start every day (as part of your morning routine) by planning out the items you'll need to complete your exercise for the day.

EXAMPLES:

- If you are going to the gym, you might need a change of clothes, a water bottle, and a yoga mat (if you do yoga).
- If you are going to be exercising outside, you might need warm clothes (if it's cold), a water bottle, running shoes, an exercise mat, a bottle of sunscreen or a hat, visor, or pair of sunglasses.
- If you are working out at home, you might need ankle weights, hand weights, an exercise mat, cardio equipment, or a workout DVD and DVD player if you are going that route.

Another idea is to store a bag in your car containing ALL the equipment you'll ever need to exercise.

For instance, I keep a "go bag" in my trunk that contains an old pair of running shoes, socks, underwear, shorts, a long-sleeved running shirt, a running singlet, a jacket, gloves, a hat, a watch, a headlamp, and a pair of spandex pants.

With this bag, I'm prepared for any type of weather (and level of light) that might occur. This completely eliminates the "I don't have the right equipment" excuse from the equation.

HOW TO IMPLEMENT

Step One:

Start out each morning (when you are at your freshest) by planning out your exercise practice for the day. Ask yourself the following questions:

- "What will my exercise be?"
- "How long will I exercise?"
- "What equipment and clothing do I need to complete my exercise?"
- "What do I need to pack with me?"

Step Two:

Be prepared with an emergency pack in your car or at your place of work that contains workout clothes, shoes, a towel, deodorant, a water bottle, and the essentials you need to complete your workout.

Step Three:

Be ready for obstacles. Remember that things won't go smoothly, so don't get discouraged and quit when you encounter an obstacle. When you already have in your mind that temptation and obstacles will come, you will be mentally prepared to overcome and push past them.

Tactic #7: Make Exercise Fun

"Boredom" is one of the biggest excuses people give for not exercising. Yes, fitness is great and you may realize the benefits, but the truth is exercise can be repetitive and not always the most enjoyable activity in the world.

Fortunately, there are many strategies you can use to fight boredom in your exercise habits:

#1. Experiment. Try different exercises until you find something that's personally enjoyable. Don't feel like you "have" an activity that you enjoy? Then keep trying different activities until you find something that works for you.

#2. Join group classes. Look for a local aerobics class. Seek out classes that are both fun and engaging. If you are a social person, this will give you the opportunity to interact with other people and build relationships while you are meeting your exercise goals. You don't have to go solo in this process of building up your good habits.

#3. Switch things up. Even if you like one particular exercise, try different activities. There may be something else out there you would enjoy even more, but you'll never know until you try.

Get out into the world and see what kinds of activities are out there that may be outside the norm. If you lift, try rock climbing. If you run, mix it up with different locations, trails, and running workouts. For example, rather than doing just sprints, hills, and distance runs, go to the beach and run in the surf, or try one of those obstacle races (like Spartan Race or Tough Mudder) that are gaining popularity.

#4. Find a new workout location. Get out of the gym on nice days. Gyms can be awesome for fitness, but sometimes being outside makes exercise more enjoyable. It can reinforce your habits and routines when you simply get out and enjoy the beautiful weather.

As an example, you can use a park bench for many of your "gym" exercises—rebounding, dips, sit-ups, and more. It can be a nice change to your routine and give you a boost in morale. Think of your favorite fitness routine and come up with ways to make it "outside" on nice days.

#5. Try a new workout machine. For example, elliptical machines can be a great break from running. Running is an excellent form of exercise, and many runners describe it as a great activity to clear your mind, but sometimes running outside can be stressful because you have to focus to avoid accidents if traffic is heavy.

Using an elliptical machine or riding a stationary bicycle, however, is a great way to completely "zone out" while exercising. You can daydream, think about solutions to your problems, read a book, watch TV, or do just about anything at all while your body exercises on autopilot.

#6. Get an education or enjoy some entertainment. Use apps such as Stitcher or iTunes to catch up on podcasts you enjoy (or discover new ones!), or work out when you know your favorite television show will be on. Most people in a gym will watch whatever happens to be on, but if you are listening to or watching your favorite programming, the time will fly by quite pleasantly.

#7. Make fitness a competition. If you have friends of similar ability and fitness level, start a friendly fitness competition with them. Try to outdo one another by achieving specific fitness goals and metrics. Even boring routines can be fun when there's a little competition to spice things up. (We'll talk more about this in the next section.)

HOW TO IMPLEMENT

Step One:

Decide which one of the seven ideas listed above you want to implement this week. Then try a different one next week.

Step Two:

Test out each idea to see how it enhances your exercise time. Are you enjoying yourself more? Still bored? If you are still experiencing boredom, try another one of the seven solutions until you find the right activities to keep you interested.

Step Three:

Don't let boredom stop you. Sometimes all we need to conquer the obstacle of boredom is a change in perspective. Is brushing your teeth boring? Yes. Do you still do it? I'd like to think so!

Some things in life may not be as exciting as you might like them to be, but when you are building life-changing, lifelong habits, it's important to just set your mind on sticking to your commitment. The great thing is that, once you have built the exercise habit, it will be much easier to keep going because it will become a part of your daily life.

Tactic #8: Take Advantage of Technology

A great way to get the motivation you need to keep working out is to track your exercise habits and compete with others. Often, this can provide that extra push when you don't feel up for exercise. A great way to do this is with apps and wearable devices that monitor your activity.

As an example, I stay motivated about my walking habit because I'm part of the <u>Fitbit community</u>. The Fitbit tracks my daily steps and ranks me versus my friends. Just that small bit of competition helps me get more movement throughout the day.

Technology can be a great thing. It can help you track, monitor, and stay up to date on all sorts of beneficial fitness stuff. Throughout the book, I will offer occasional tech solutions for specific problems and ideas. Understand that these ideas are just a *sample* of many of the great devices that are available to fitness aficionados.

HOW TO IMPLEMENT

Just about any fitness-related problem has a tech solution that will, at a minimum, help with the situation. Here is just a small sampling of some of the tech stuff out there:

- Heart rate monitors
- Activity monitors (Fitbit: iTunes, Google Play)
- Chains.cc (iTunes)
- Coach.me (iTunes, Google Play)
- Pace/elevation watches (Fitbit Surge or Garmin Forerunner)
- Walking desks (LifeSpan or TrekDesk)
- The top "wearable devices" (Polar FT4 Heart Rate Monitor)
- You can even put money on the line with an app like Fitsby.
- Exercise logs (like the Runner's Log app)

- Podrunner: Set the intensity of your workout (135 heartbeats per minute, 160 bpm, etc.); then download music that matches it.

You can also turn your workout into a game. Many apps and personal fitness trackers are beginning to gamify the workout process. Here are some examples:

- For walking, check out Ingress (iTunes, Google Play) to hack some aliens or The Walk (iTunes, Google Play) to find yourself fighting the enemy during wartime in the UK.
- For running, fight zombies with Zombies, Run! (iTunes, Google Play), get into a sci-fi adventure with BattleSuit Runner Fitness (iTunes, Google Play) or see what it's like to run the Boston Marathon with the Virtual Runner app.
- For strength training, use the app Adventure Workout on Google Play, and have fun battling ogres, werewolves, and goblins.

As you can see, there is a veritable goldmine of apps and devices that help you stay competitive when it comes to exercise. Many of them have a built-in level of social engagement so you can create challenges with friends and acquaintances. This taps into one of the most powerful motivational tools—accountability. Let's talk about that next.

Tactic #9: Be Accountable

A way to supercharge your motivation and solidify your commitment is to join forces with others and enlist their help. Studies have shown that having accountability when trying to make lifestyle changes (including exercise) has a positive, long-term impact.

There's a principle called the Hawthorne effect (or observer effect) that came from a series of experiments from the 1920s. The studies revealed that when people were being observed, they wanted to look good and perform well. They were more likely to give more effort if they were being watched.

The Hawthorne effect shows us that, to improve our chances of success, we must put ourselves out there to be observed by others. While tracking and monitoring with devices and apps *can help*, when you put yourself in a position to get both positive and negative feedback on a habit, you're more likely to follow through on a daily basis.

Accountability is a critical part of habit development—whether you are trying to change a bad habit or reinforce a good one. The only danger with accountability is if you are too competitive and push yourself too hard to the point of injury or burnout. However, this should not stop you from being accountable to someone. Just be cognizant of this danger if you are hyper-competitive.

As part of the exercise habit mentality, your accountability needs to focus on meeting your specific goals. Let those micro-commitments guide you and keep you from going overboard. Be satisfied with what you have accomplished each day you complete your exercise goal, understand what you are capable of doing, and stick to those boundaries until your body and mind are ready to take things a step further.

HOW TO IMPLEMENT

Step One:

Share your goal with others. Whether it is family members, friends, co-workers, or people you meet through an online forum, you need to have someone (or more than one person) who will listen to you explain your goals and your plan for achieving your goals.

You can even find a "check-in buddy"—someone you regularly talk to and share your successes and failures with. It works even better if this person is also into regular exercise; this way, you can support each other. No matter who you partner with for accountability, be sure to include deadlines for milestones and regular updates so you can keep the accountability going.

Step Two:

Go public. Share your goals via your social media profiles or on other online forums to get encouragement and accountability. You can even publish a video diary on YouTube, or start your own blog to share the details of what you are doing with the purpose of connecting with other people. You can also turn to apps suggested in prior sections of this book to get some extra accountability.

Step Three:

Connect with people in real life. Go to MeetUp.com and look for local groups related to health and fitness.

Can't find one? Then start a new group! You may be surprised by how scheduling something in your area could meet a big need for many people. Being able to meet once a week, every other week, or even once a month could help you to establish some solid accountability.

Step Four:

If you are having trouble finding someone to provide the accountability you need to succeed, consider hiring a personal trainer or coach. This will be someone who can be right beside you, offering suggestions and feedback to help you meet your goals.

Step Five:

Sign a contract with yourself. This will formalize your goals into specific results and measurable metrics, which helps you treat this "idea" of regular exercise as a formal agreement. Just having something formal makes you more likely to be successful.

The website StickK.com offers an excellent tool for creating a contract. You can even put money on the line!

For example, find a family member or friend with some philosophical viewpoints that differ from yours. Then, ask them to name a charity you may not like (to make the donation painful). An example would be the National Rifle Association (NRA) if you dislike guns. If you break your contract, you have to donate to this cause.

Get creative and have fun. Use whatever it takes to stick to your goals.

Tactic #10: Overcome Lack of Results

Let's face it, seeing a "lack of results" can be the ultimate motivation killer.

You might say to yourself, *"I worked out for 20 days but didn't lose any weight, so honestly, why do I even bother?"*

It's easy to get discouraged when you're not hitting your goals like you anticipated. Trust me, you're not the only person who looks in the mirror after the first workout and expects to see a noticeable difference. There's just something wired into our brains to make us think we need to see immediate results.

Don't let a lack of immediate results prevent you from experiencing the long-term benefits of building the exercise habit. Remember, the ultimate goal is to create a new daily routine. This is something you won't immediately see in the mirror or on the scale.

It's important to understand three core things about exercising:

#1. Muscle is denser and heavier than fat. When you exercise a lot and burn more calories than you consume, you are building muscle *and* burning fat. While your fat may be decreasing, your heavier muscle may be increasing for little net change in weight.

#2. Denser muscle will burn calories while doing nothing, and with time and effort, your weight will go down.

#3. In the beginning stages of this process, you may not *see* any difference on the scale after eating healthier and exercising, but that doesn't mean there are no results. You need to give it time. Plus, you should keep track of specific metrics like waist size and how your clothes are fitting instead of just tracking a number on the scale.

To get past those demotivating moments where you're not seeing the results as quickly as you want, you should take time to explore other aspects of your life to see if you might be sabotaging your efforts.

For example, if you are building the exercise habit but still eating poorly, you may be negating your efforts. While your primary focus now is to build the exercise habit, it's important to be aware of factors like sleep and nutrition because it all plays into your results.

HOW TO IMPLEMENT

If you're not getting the "results" that you would like to see, then you might want to consider the following:

Step One:

Analyze your eating habits. If you exercise just for weight loss, your time would be better spent focusing on modifying your eating habits (and this doesn't mean simply dieting). You should control portion sizes and focus on what you're eating. Then, once that is in place, start adding in more exercise.

If you reward yourself with food after workouts, then this might be preventing you from losing weight. For example, burning 500 calories during exercise and then "treating" yourself to a McDonald's cheeseburger means you just ate nearly as much as you burned.

Step Two:

Consider your exercise activity. Are you doing enough to achieve the results you desire? Of course, any workout is better than nothing, but if you want results, you sometimes have to push yourself a bit.

For instance, walking for 15 minutes a day is a positive action, but don't expect magical results in the weight-loss department if that's all the daily exercise you get. It's a great place to start, but you may need to push it to see results. However, for the purposes of your 30-day process of building the exercise habit, it's important to focus more on the goal of consistency than it is to go overboard exercising to achieve weight-loss goals.

Step Three:

Determine if you are doing too much too soon. If you are overly tired, constantly in pain or have trouble completing workouts, you're probably doing too much. Truthfully, going overboard with exercising causes your muscles to constantly break down and often leads to burnout.

Step Four:

Assess the type of workout you are doing. Are you incorporating both aerobic and anaerobic exercise? Aerobic means "with oxygen," while anaerobic means "without oxygen." Weight loss requires a mixture of both.

Aerobic exercise is when you get your heart rate up but can still hold a conversation while working out. It's good for burning lots of calories to take off the fat.

Anaerobic exercise is the type where you get out of breath in just a few moments, like during a sprint or when you are quickly climbing stairs. It builds muscle mass, which helps you burn more calories more efficiently when you exercise and even when you sit around.

If weight loss is your goal, vary your routine so you incorporate both aerobic and anaerobic exercises.

Step Five:

Check your expectations. You may simply be expecting too much too soon. Weight loss, exercise, and fitness are best handled as a lifelong process.

With the popularity of Atkins, South Beach, the hCG diet, fasting, and super-low-calorie diets, people often expect amazing results quickly. Healthy, lasting weight loss doesn't work like this. The right kind of fitness, weight loss, and nutrition takes a long time to come about. It took a long time to put on weight, so it will take a while to take it off.

This book is not about weight loss, but if you want to do it right, you will need to create a lifelong habit of exercise *and* sensible eating. What's important to remember is it will take time to see results on the scale.

Tactic #11: Relate Exercise to a Goal

> *"A goal is a dream with a deadline."*
> — Napoleon Hill

A great way to be motivated to exercise every day is to tie the habit to a short-term (or even a lifelong) goal. Goals take an intangible idea and set a plan for making it real. Without this plan, your fitness dreams will be almost impossible to achieve.

As an example, I've already mentioned that one of my core exercise goals is running marathons. One reason I stick to this habit is because I have a **lifelong goal** of completing a marathon in each state in the U.S. That's a total of 50 total marathons.

I stay motivated because there's always another marathon on the horizon. For instance, as I write these words, I'm preparing for the Salt Lake City race (Utah, April 2015), and I've already registered for the Chicago Marathon in the fall (Illinois, October 2015).

Never underestimate the power of setting goals. This can be your sole motivation for those times when you're tired and not in the mood to exercise. Goals are often the answer to that nagging question that pops into your mind: *"What's the point of exercising today?"*

The key to effective goal setting is to clearly define your anticipated outcomes. My preferred method is to do it in the S.M.A.R.T. format *(Specific, Measurable, Attainable, Relevant, and Time-Bound)*.

It isn't enough to say, *"I want to be rich."* This vague statement doesn't say anything about *how* and *when* you will achieve the outcome. In fact, it doesn't even clarify what you mean by the term "rich" or what, according to you, is "poor."

You can't create an action plan if you don't have a clear description of your desired outcome.

The solution?

Use **S.M.A.R.T.** goals.

Here is a breakdown of what this means.

S: Specific

Answer six "W" questions in relation to your goal: *who, what, where, when, which* and *why*.

When you can identify each element, you will know which actions are required to reach your goal. Specificity is important because when you reach these milestones (date, location, and objective), you'll know for certain you have achieved your goal.

M: Measurable

Define your goal with precise times, amounts, weights, measurements, blood test numbers, or anything that measures progress toward your goal. Creating measurable goals makes it easy to determine if you have progressed from point A to point B. Measurable goals also help you figure out when you're headed in the right direction and when you're not.

A: Attainable

This aspect stretches the limits of what you think is possible. While these goals are not impossible to complete, they're often challenging and full of obstacles. The key to creating an attainable goal is to look at your current life and set an objective that seems *slightly* beyond your reach. That way, even if you fail, you still accomplish something of significance.

R: Relevant

These goals focus on what you truly desire. They are the exact opposite of inconsistent or scattered goals. They are in harmony with everything that is important in your life, from success in your career to happiness with the people you love.

T: Time-Bound

These goals have specific deadlines. You are expected to achieve your desired outcome before a target date. Time-bound goals are challenging and grounding. The key to creating a time-bound goal is to set a deadline you'll meet by working backward and developing new habits.

S.M.A.R.T. goals are clear and well defined. There is no doubt about the result you want to achieve. At its deadline, you'll know if you *have* or *haven't* achieved a particular goal.

HOW TO IMPLEMENT

Step One:

Create a series of S.M.A.R.T. goals that includes both short-term goals (deadlines within three months) and long-term goals (any time after that). With the long-term goals, the sky is the limit. Even if you fail in "reaching for the stars," you may well reach the "moon," which, in terms of exercise, will help you achieve significant results. The key is to focus on incremental goals.

For example, slowly increase the length and intensity of your exercise sessions. Walk before you run (literally and figuratively).

You can have very lofty goals. Sure, you can intend to run marathons, even if you don't currently run at all, but the first steps should be short jogs or long walks. Then, build up to doing 1 to 2 miles. Then, a 5K race. Then, a 10K race. Then, a half-marathon. Then, finally, train for a marathon. Depending on your fitness level, this may take years of work, so don't be discouraged by not doing enough in the early stages.

Step Two:

Understand what outcome you want from exercise: *Weight loss? Fun? Community? Train for a big event (like a marathon)? Bulk up? Live longer?* Keep in mind that people overestimate what they can do in the short term and underestimate what can be done on a long-term basis.

For the short term, your plan should be reasonable and actionable. Stick to easily achievable goals and don't forget to have fun! For the long term, the sky is the limit. What is your dream? If you can dream it, you can do it.

Step Three:

Set a <u>specific</u> start date, but only after preparing physically and mentally for obstacles and identifying triggers. This may mean that you don't rush out and immediately start exercising. This isn't to say you can't go out and exercise right away if you feel like it, but tell yourself those exercise days won't count for routine-building purposes. Every new habit needs a firm start date, or you'll keep pushing it off.

Step Four:

Make your exercise goals measurable: three sets of 30 sit-ups, a 1-mile walk, or a 15-minute jog. There should be a specific number attached to all goals—either time or quantity.

As a reminder, when starting out, make these goals as simple as possible—consistency and streaking are more important than a specific number. It will be important to get a baseline metric so you know where you are starting and can gauge your progress.

Step Five:

Write down your goals and review them regularly. It is important to put these written goals somewhere you can see them. Whether it's by your computer monitor, inside a mobile app, or posted near your calendar, keep your goals in view. This will help you to maintain your focus, even when distractions come your way.

OBSTACLE (3):
MENTAL STUMBLING BLOCKS

> *"Whether you think you can, or you think you can't—you're right."*
> – Henry Ford

Many people beat themselves up because they don't exercise. If you believe you can't do something, you won't.

It goes something like this:

Negative mindset → Negative beliefs → Negative behaviors → Negative results

See how that works?

The same is true for having a positive mindset. Stay positive and the positive results will follow. Sure, you are going to have a negative mindset from time to time. When you get a ticket on your way to work, get the flu, or see your child's crummy report card, you are going to feel negative. If you have 50 things that go well in a day and one thing that goes wrong, human nature is to focus on that one bad thing.

When it comes to exercise, you <u>will</u> feel negative at times, but you have to find a way to let go of these feelings and focus on the results you're moving toward. It takes practice, though. It won't come naturally for most people. You will have to be mindful and use positive self-talk to redirect your thoughts from negative to positive. Just like you are building your daily exercise habit, you may have to start building your positive thinking habit.

Let's take a look at some solutions for overcoming negative thoughts and the mental stumbling blocks you might encounter along the way.

Tactic #12: Realign Your Notion of "Exercise"

People are very rigid with their thinking of what constitutes "exercise." Thanks to the marketing of fitness and weight-loss products, we are bombarded by messages about how only one brand of fitness is the best way to stay in shape.

It's important to keep a proper perspective and understand that behind this message of "this is the *best workout* to use if you want to look like this" is a company trying to sell you something. Their goal is to make you believe that, if you want to succeed, you need to exercise their way.

This is simply a lie. You don't need the latest, greatest fitness DVD on the market to develop the exercise habit. You don't even have to use it to meet your ultimate fitness or weight-loss goals.

Any type of consistent, active movement is exercise.

That's right…ANY type of movement is considered exercising your body. Whether it is cleaning your house vigorously, walking to the mailbox, dancing in the kitchen with your kids, or going up and down stairs as you put away laundry—it's all exercise.

Really, if you a stick to an activity that raises your pulse, produces sweat, and can be done on a consistent basis, then (in my opinion) that's good enough to be considered exercise.

HOW TO IMPLEMENT

Step One:

Tune out the marketing messages, or at least see them for what they really are—a way to make you feel that you <u>need</u> specific products to experience fulfillment.

Once you've gained perspective on these messages in our culture, on television, and on social media, you will find they hold much less power over you. They no longer define for you what exercise is, which paves the way for a much healthier, realistic perspective that you can use to build the exercise habit.

Step Two:

Continually remind yourself that ANY movement is a form of exercise, and then find ways to work a variety of movement into your day. Some examples might be:

- Doing squats as you brush your teeth.
- Jogging to the mailbox and then around the block before you come back home.
- More squats while doing the dishes.
- Walking the half mile to the convenience store instead of driving.
- Dancing with the kids (or by yourself) after dinner.
- Stretching periodically during your workday.
- Taking the stairs at the office.
- Parking at the farthest spot from the door when you make your grocery run.
- Doing jumping jacks during advertisements as you watch your favorite show.

While setting aside a specific time for your fitness habit is important, finding opportunities to work in movement when you can will enhance your results. Plus, it reinforces the idea that exercise is not just what the media tells you it is. Instead, it's something you can do throughout the day.

Tactic #13: Stop Being Obsessed with Goals

Okay, I know…this strategy contradicts the section where talked about the importance of setting goals. However (in my opinion), there is a fine line between being goal-*oriented* and goal-*obsessed*.

Goals are powerful things in fitness. Everyone should have goals; however, like anything else, too much of a good thing can have a detrimental impact.

Being too goal-oriented can make it all about competition and winning—in both formal competitions and beating personal bests. Having this obsession to win and succeed can lead to:

- Stress
- Anger
- Loss of self-worth

These are not feelings you want to create in your life.

Let's take a look at an example:

Two runners train, enter a race, and cross the finish line. The goal-obsessed runner is upset because he didn't win or even place in the race. The goal-oriented runner has a healthier perspective and knows that she did her best. This runner understands the race is a part of the process on the way to reaching long-term goals.

Obsession rarely ends well because it's never enough. You can't do enough or be enough, so you continually feel like you are falling short, or you may feel like a complete failure. This is a dangerous place to be.

The goal-obsessed person is also likely to be so laser-focused on a certain goal that once it *is* achieved, he just drops it and completely stops the practice. This obviously doesn't help to create the lifelong exercise habit.

The key is to find that healthy balance. You need goals in your life, but you don't need obsession. If you feel yourself becoming obsessed and nothing else is as important as your goal, it's time to pause and reevaluate why you started this process.

For instance, I previously mentioned that I use the Fitbit to monitor my daily steps. One feature of this device is your friends can "taunt" you or challenge you to various fitness challenges. While I do my best to participate, I never allow competition to morph into an obsession. If I know I've exercised enough for the week, then I simply ignore these messages instead of falling into the trap of pushing myself too much (and potentially causing an injury).

Taking a look at the "bigger picture" and focusing on long-term goals can help you to recapture a healthier perspective and achieve the balance you need to make this experience as positive and beneficial as possible.

HOW TO IMPLEMENT

Step One:

Check yourself before you wreck yourself.

If you feel like your goal-oriented nature is bordering on obsessive behavior, it's time to do some self-analysis and mental regrouping. Goals are important and good, but it is the process that truly matters. It goes along with the idea that you can't see the forest for the trees. I want you to be able to get that big-picture perspective so you see the trees *and* the forest.

Step Two:

Your primary goal needs to stay the same: create the daily exercise habit.

The reason I keep saying this is because it's the whole purpose of this book.

Even if you have big fitness, weight-loss, or performance goals, it's the small steps that will establish a solid foundation for your health. Without this foundation, it'll be really difficult to achieve your long-term goals because you'll either burn out from pushing too hard or give up altogether.

Tactic #14: Overcome Plateaus

The issue of plateaus is especially a concern for those exercising solely for weight loss, bulking up, and participating in competitions. The truth is, there *will* come a time when repeating the same routine won't yield the progressive results you once saw. In fact, you might even see a *decrease* in results.

If this happens, don't panic.

Here's why: It takes the body about 4 to 6 weeks to adapt to a new workout.

When the body adapts to the new regimen, it will become more efficient, consuming less energy, using fewer calories, and storing less fat. You may not see the fat burn and the drop in weight like you experienced in the beginning, but remember that this is normal and to be expected.

Many people get discouraged during their plateaus. Often, they feel like they're doing something wrong. Some even make the mistake of increasing the intensity of their workouts.

Unfortunately, this tactic can quickly become an arms race that goes against the "Exercise Every Day" philosophy.

Unless you want exercise to be the dominant focus of your life, the best strategy for overcoming plateaus is to mix up your daily routine.

As a runner, this could mean adding hills to a daily run or adding in sprint intervals. It could also mean trying different exercises. You could try swimming once a week or a CrossFit class. Whatever you decide to do, mix it up in order to keep your body guessing.

One reason people love CrossFit is they rarely go through the same workout. Each day comes with a new set of exercises and challenges. People who do CrossFit don't hit plateaus because they're constantly testing (and exhausting) different muscle groups.

Another thing you can do to break through a plateau is to **forget about weight loss**. I realize this is easier said than done, but if you're always worried about losing weight, you won't have the mental fortitude to get through those rough patches. The important thing to remember is that if you eat less and exercise more, the weight loss will almost always come eventually.

HOW TO IMPLEMENT

Step One:

Understand that plateaus will come. They are a normal part of the process of increasing your fitness level or losing weight. If you can get your mind set on the idea of plateaus, you will be able to deal with them in a healthier way when they come (and face a lot less frustration). Just like you prepare yourself for other exercise obstacles, being prepared for plateaus will set you up for success in the long term.

Step Two:

Mix it up when the plateaus come. When you start to see diminishing results, add in a few new exercises. If you are a runner, throw in some swimming or lifting. If you do a particular home workout DVD, try something different. The idea is to keep your body guessing.

Step Three:

Focus on the long-term goal of establishing a solid exercise habit. When you take the focus off of weight loss, a particular clothing size, or a number on the scale, you will take a lot of pressure off yourself. You will also find yourself enjoying the process more.

If you continue to work out daily and keep your nutrition in check, the results will come in time. If weight loss is one of your goals, check your metrics no more than once a week. Once a month might be even better; it is reasonable to expect a loss in that amount of time.

Tactic #15: Deal with Your Self-Consciousness

A major mental stumbling block is when you feel like you're being judged by others.

Perhaps you're scared to go to the gym or perform your exercise outside where people can see you.

Maybe you are overweight and feel insecure about how you appear working out with all of the extra weight on your body.

I often hear this from people.

You may experience feelings of despair and insecurity or find yourself continually comparing yourself with others who are fit and lean.

You may feel intimidated by sports stores, gyms, personal trainers, and other people in the fitness world.

I get it.

It can seem overwhelming and scary when you are not used to this culture. It's a new and foreign environment for those who are not used to fitness. (We'll talk more about how to handle working out in a gym later in the book.) Any time you try something new, there is a period of insecurity and uneasiness.

This is NORMAL.

YOU are normal for feeling this way.

However, if left unchecked, these fears can hold you back, limit your exercise routines, and keep you from becoming fit.

The reality?

Most people are self-centered.

They're in their own world. They don't care about your fitness and won't waste time judging you. (And if they do, they are jerks, and you don't want those people in your life.)

In fact, if anything, there is a sense of community when seeing someone making an effort. Given a chance, most people who are into fitness would be more likely to help and support than to judge, so don't assume people are thinking the worst of you.

And what if someone does judge you or makes you feel out of place? Does it really matter? Are you going to let some judgmental jerk keep you from meeting your goals to improve your life?

No way!

Your health and well-being are far too important. You have set goals that are important to you. Any time you put yourself out there to make a change in life, there *will* be people who want to pass judgment and bring you down. Usually, it is because of their own personal problems or hard times. It's more about them than it is about you, so pay them no attention and get on with your bad self!

HOW TO IMPLEMENT

Step One:

Choose the right place to work out. While you should not feel a need to hide in your basement and exercise away from the rest of the world, jumping right into the middle of your local gym may not be the best answer for you either.

Start your fitness routine in an area where you are comfortable. Women may feel more comfortable in all-female gyms. Those who are overweight may feel more comfortable in programs with others who are struggling with their weight. If you're extremely self-conscious, pick a gym that isn't that crowded or go at off-peak times.

As an example, the entire marketing campaign of <u>Planet Fitness</u> revolves around providing members with a "Judgment-Free Zone." While this gym might not be in your area, others have started to recognize the importance of creating a comfortable workout environment. My advice? Look for this type of gym in your area.

Step Two:

Get some support.

If you do go to a gym, or even want to exercise outside, getting a coach or personal trainer can make the process easier. With a personal trainer, the fear of doing exercises "wrong" or using improper form goes away. Taking the time to get educated on your specific fitness goals can build self-confidence.

Even an exercise buddy can help. Having someone else to work out with will keep you from feeling self-conscious and alone. It's hard to feel as isolated and out of place when you have someone else exercising with you.

Step Three:

Lose yourself and get in the zone so you aren't paying attention to those around you. Put on headphones, watch TV while exercising (at the gym), or read a book on a stationary bike. If you occupy your mind while working out, many of the feelings of self-consciousness will disappear.

Tactic #16: Deal with Self-Sabotage

The truth is we are often our own worst enemies. There's that little voice in your head giving you many reasons not to do things. The reasons for this often boil down to insecurity, fear, and procrastination.

It's pretty easy to make excuses to self-sabotage our best-laid plans. It's important to know when these excuses are *valid* and when they *prevent you from taking action*. When you are making a big life change, it's common to have a part of you resist the efforts. This is due to some self-limiting beliefs or fears you may not even realize you have.

When you can take some time to explore what is behind your excuses and self-sabotaging efforts, you will be able to get past them and move on to taking the action necessary to achieve your goals.

Let's take a look at **seven of the most common self-limiting beliefs, doubts, and questions** you may have and discuss the root problem behind each one.

#1—How do I know my plan will work?

With so many plans and programs out there claiming to be the only way to succeed in fitness or weight loss, it is easy to start wondering how your plan can work. It comes back to focusing on your fitness plan and nothing else until you get it down. Unless you are committed to doing your plan and building a foundation of solid exercise habits, you will find yourself with "shiny object syndrome," always looking for the next great thing and never really taking action.

#2—It doesn't matter.

When you feel overwhelmed by the challenges of life, you may find yourself thinking that this exercise stuff doesn't matter. One of the simplest remedies to the "doesn't matter" excuse is to simply focus on your level of consistency. That's it. Remind yourself that daily action is all you need to do, nothing more.

#3—I have failed at this so many times already.

Believing you are a failure is a major self-limiting belief. If you let it go unchecked, it can hold you back in all areas of your life. You must know that we all fail. Every single person. The difference between the people who eventually find success and the ones who don't is that the successful ones pick themselves back up and keep going after the failures. The fact that you have failed in the past means nothing other than that you are a human being.

#4—This takes too much time.

Sure, this is a valid excuse. Adding exercise to your life requires a time commitment. But everyone is busy, and yet many people still find time to create exercise habits; you can, too.

The "no time" excuse is another one of those things that can hold you back in all areas of your life if you let it. Subconsciously, many people make this excuse with the secret hope that the need to do the task will eventually disappear. The need to develop an exercise habit to keep yourself healthy is never going to go away. You know that. So don't let this excuse hold you down any longer.

#5—I don't feel like it today.

Why do you not want to exercise? Is it a fear of failure? Discomfort? Or just lack of interest?

The good news is that whatever is behind your lack of desire is basically remedied with the strategies described in this book.

You don't have to commit to hours of exercise—just enough movement to meet your goal.

You don't have to be in pain or set yourself up for failure— you have chosen a workout plan that fits your unique fitness level and goals.

You don't have to deal with a boring workout.

Throughout this book, you'll learn a number of options to help you mix it up and keep things fun and interesting.

#6—I keep forgetting.

This is often subconscious avoidance. People often procrastinate on a task because they "forget" to do it. Sure, we all have those moments when something honestly slips our minds. However, being chronically forgetful is a sign of a deep-seated resistance toward a specific task.

Perhaps you don't think it's important. Maybe you're scared of failure. Or perhaps you're not using an effective organizational system. The point here is that "forgetting" isn't a valid reason for procrastination.

You can beat this issue by scheduling MANY reminders. Set reminders on your smartphone alarm, or check out these apps with built-in workout reminders to help you remember your commitment:

- Workout Trainer (iTunes, Google Play, Kindle)
- Body-weight Training (iTunes, Google Play)
- Daily Workouts (iTunes, Google Play, Kindle)
- Pushups Trainer (iTunes)
- Coco's Workout World (iTunes)

#7—I need to do X first, or I will do it after this event/date.

There's always some reason to put things off, isn't there? The same thing is true for working out. You might think you will get started with your workout program after you have accomplished certain tasks or after you get some project, event, or date out of the way, but something is bound to crop up.

This is real life—you'll never have a blank schedule.

Don't let the fairy tale idea of needing "more free time" keep you from working out. Your schedule is probably never going to be perfectly clear. After all, you are an adult with adult responsibilities, so just get committed to incorporating your daily exercise habit, no matter what other things are going on in your life.

HOW TO IMPLEMENT

Step One:

Take time to write out your personal self-sabotage excuses. Knowing what excuses you tend to use gives you the power to recognize the excuse for what it is when it comes around. You can refer to the list above to give yourself the positive self-talk you need to break through self-sabotaging tendencies.

Step Two:

When you feel like you are constantly getting bombarded by excuses, stay focused on your fitness commitment and nothing more. This habit takes up little time, is painless, and is customized to your needs and interests, so reminding yourself of this commitment will help you stay on track.

OBSTACLE (4):
NOT ENOUGH TIME

Isn't life *crazy busy?*
You have work, the daily commute, kids, the carpool, extended family obligations, and extra-curricular activities, and that doesn't even count time for hobbies and entertainment. At times, it seems impossible to include those "extras" in your life. There are days when you think it is simply too much to even try to squeeze in your exercise.

Am I right?

The way to get around this is to stop viewing exercise as an optional activity. It should *never* be in the same category as catching a movie or getting your nails done. This is serious business that will impact the quality of your life, your health, and your well-being.

For this reason, you need to schedule your exercise time like an appointment with your boss. It's not always easy or what you want to do, but you'd better show up.

If you are an entrepreneur (like I am) or have a day full of intense work, there can be too much focus on business, making it hard to shut down for the day.

Instead of seeing exercise as an inconvenience, you must reframe your perspective and begin viewing it as an opportunity to release stress, get energized, and gain clarity on your workday. In fact, working out will increase your productivity, enhance your stamina, and decrease your stress levels so you can be a better employee or business owner.

See what I did there?

I used a principle called "reframing" to show how exercise can positively impact other areas of your life.

Reframing is very powerful and enables you to take an entirely new approach. By doing this, you can begin thinking about your fitness habit as a way to enhance your life, rather than as an annoying time-sucker.

Let's talk about a few strategies to help you find time for this important habit.

Tactic #17: Get More Time

You've heard it said before:

"We all have the same 24 hours in a day; it's what you do with them that counts."

There is always time in your day, but how you choose to use it will determine whether or not you achieve your goals.

If you feel like you are continually short on time and unable to exercise, there is a serious question you need to ask yourself: *How badly do you want to meet your goals? Are you willing to sacrifice something in order to meet them?*

If you determine that you do have a desire to meet your goals and will do what it takes to make your daily exercise practice happen, then exercise must become a top priority.

This means it comes before entertainment, pleasure, extra sleep, or chatting with friends. You do what it takes, just like you do what it takes to make sure the oil gets changed in your car or that you brush your teeth each day.

Here are some ideas for activities you can cut down on to free up time for your exercise habit:

- Checking email
- Using social media (FB, Twitter, Instagram, Pinterest)
- Reading
- Watching TV
- Internet browsing
- Going to manicure/massage/salon appointments
- Flat-ironing or curling your hair (wear it in an easier style)
- Keeping your house spic-and-span (I'm not saying let things get filthy; just don't worry about keeping it in a perfect, clutter-free state every waking moment.)

If you take the time to really assess how you spend the minutes and hours of your day, you can, without a doubt, find ways to free up more time, even if it's just 15 or 20 minutes a day in 5-

minute increments. You'll discover there are activities you can eliminate if you are willing to make some small sacrifices.

HOW TO IMPLEMENT

Step One:

Spend a week tracking the time you spend on all activities throughout the day. Make a spreadsheet or just write it down in a notebook, but physically track what you are doing, the time of day you are doing it, and the amount of time it takes. Be detailed and account for even the small things in your day.

Step Two:

Use the Rescue Time app to monitor what you do online. It will keep a log of all the sites you visit and how long you are there. No, you really don't need to spend 45 minutes a day watching BuzzFeed videos or keeping tabs on what every single friend on Facebook is doing.

Step Three:

Once you have accounted for your time, start marking off the unessential tasks. By eliminating 15 minutes on Twitter, 30 minutes on Facebook, and 45 minutes watching videos, for example, you have a very nice amount of time in which you can incorporate your daily exercise habit.

With this three-step process, you might not even feel the pain of sacrifice because you aren't cutting out essential tasks in your day. It's just extra fluff and time-wasters that really add very little value to your life. Also, nothing says you can't check Facebook or watch a few videos while you are on the treadmill.

Tactic #18: Maximize Small Pockets of Time

This is the perfect strategy for the super-busy person reading this book. (You know who you are.)

Even when you cut your activities to the bare essentials, you may still find it hard to find large amounts of uninterrupted time to devote to your exercise habit.

That's okay!

Remember, we aren't doing all-or-nothing thinking here; we are building a habit that will (hopefully) fit into your hectic lifestyle for years to come. If you are a busy person, you can make this work by maximizing small pockets of time within your packed schedule.

One of the reasons I like activity trackers (like the Fitbit) is because they count steps. So instead of committing to 30 minutes each day, you make micro-commitments to get up and move around as often as you can...even if it is for 5 minutes here and there.

These 5- to 10-minute pockets of exercise, a few times each day, can easily add up to 30 minutes or more of exercise time.

HOW TO IMPLEMENT

If you feel you simply have too much to do every day, then consider a few creative strategies or steps to get more exercise.

Step One:

Use workout reminder apps, such as <u>Mind Jogger</u>, to help you remember to work in a bit of exercise, even if you are focused on work-related tasks. If you are experiencing a busy season at work, it's easy to lose track of time. Before you know it, you've worked at your desk for the past eight hours.

Reminders from apps can get you moving, whether it is just stretching in your cubicle or taking a walk up and down the stairs. These apps are ideal for people who are very focused on productivity and hate having to take time away from working to exercise.

Step Two:

Buy a Fitbit or other movement counter to track your steps. Then, create a small goal (like 5,000 steps) and use your short breaks to get at least a little bit of movement.

Set a reminder or alarm notifying you to take a 5-minute break every hour and use that time to walk around your office space. Walk the FULL 5 minutes. Doing this would result in 40 minutes of light exercise in an average workday…Not bad!

Another thing you can do to increase movement is take the stairs rather than using elevators at work. Do this any time you need to go up or down fewer than five floors.

Step Three:

Incorporate movement into activities you already have to do (or want to do) in your day.

For example:

- Get exercise while you work or watch television with a TrekDesk or a stationary bicycle.
- Bike to work. Anyone can bike to work in nearly any city. Check out this blog series from Mr. Money Mustache that covers how to bike to work safely and efficiently.
- Use the 7-Minute Workout app to get in a small amount of exercise first thing in the morning before you even start your day. Everyone can wake up just 7 minutes earlier, right? Let's talk about this some more with the next solution…

You'd be surprised that, with a little planning, you can easily add more movement throughout your day.

Tactic #19: Exercise in the Early Morning

Sure, it's not fun to get up early in the morning to do your workout, but you may find that creating this habit is your secret weapon for incorporating exercise into your day. You don't have to wake up 2 hours earlier to squeeze in some exercise.

Thirty minutes, 20 minutes or even just 7 minutes with the 7-Minute Workout app (for iOS) can help you meet your exercise goal, which helps you to turn it into a lifetime habit.

Right now, it might seem impossible to add more to your morning routine because—let's face it—you're already a busy person. You may characterize yourself as a night owl and just can't imagine waking up earlier to exercise.

Here's the thing, though…

I've discovered several things about mornings that have convinced me this is the perfect time of the day for self-improvement activities, including exercise.

Here are three reasons why exercising in the morning may be the perfect solution to your "not enough time" obstacle:

1. The first 30 minutes of your day will give you energy that will set the tone and help you succeed for the rest of the day.
2. If you devote your early mornings to your exercise habit, you will be less likely to skip it altogether.
3. By focusing on exercise in the morning, you will naturally work it into the rest of your day. Your energy level will be higher, and you will begin to enjoy and even crave more movement throughout your day.

Just give it a shot and see how it energizes you and helps you to work in your exercise habit more efficiently and consistently. Commit to doing it for at least a week and see what happens.

Of course, I'm not going to leave you hanging, so let's cover some real ways to implement this solution in the mornings.

HOW TO IMPLEMENT

Step One:

Decide what time you need to wake up in the morning. In order to make this work, you should plan your schedule by "reverse engineering" your day.

Start by asking these questions:

- What time do you need to drive the kids to school?
- What time to you need to be at work?
- How long does it take you to get ready in the morning?
- How long does it take to drive to work?

Once you've answered these questions, use the answers to determine how much time you need to accomplish all of these things. Then add in the extra time required to squeeze in your morning exercise.

We are starting small to create your exercise habit, so this shouldn't be a significantly earlier wake-up time, just enough to incorporate your 15-, 20- or 30-minute practice.

Step 2:

Be prepared and plan ahead. Without a plan, you will get frustrated and want to give up.

Time yourself doing your exercises so you know exactly how much time it will take. When you are timing yourself, include any set-up time as well as the time it takes for you to clean up afterward.

For instance, if you need a mat, gym clothes, or other equipment, have it all set out and ready to use the night before. Schedule your every move for the morning so you don't cut yourself too short on time and add unnecessary stress to your day.

Being prepared will make this new habit easier to incorporate and establish.

Step 3:

Keep your morning exercise session brief (especially in the beginning). It's unreasonable to think that you can suddenly wake up three hours earlier each morning and do a super-long workout. That's a fast way to burn out and want to quit before you get started.

Start small with your micro-commitments to exercise. Don't try to do more in the beginning. We are building a foundation for a lifelong habit, not preparing you for a fitness competition.

To establish the routine, you will need to:

(I.) Alter your bedtime routine to set you up for a pleasant morning and easier wake-up. If getting to sleep at a decent time is difficult for you, try to establish a soothing bedtime routine to get you ready for slumber.

(II.) Turn off your electronics one hour before bed. Remove all lights from your bedroom. Play soft music. Do whatever you need to do to create a good environment for sleeping so you can get 8 hours, if possible.

(III.) Get up earlier once you've grown accustomed to this new wake-up time.

(IV.) Add in the micro-commitment of exercise until it is a habit—a minimum of 30 days—before adding in more time for additional workouts.

You'll find that once you've adjusted your evening routine and gotten used to waking up a little earlier, you'll have the energy to engage in an enjoyable exercise routine.

Tactic #20: Exercise in the Early Evening

Exercising in the evening might not seem all that appealing to you. After all, you are hungry, tired, and simply tapped out after a stressful and busy day. Maybe you are thinking to yourself, *"I've busted my butt for the last 10 hours, so why should I do more?"* After a long, hard day, the only thing you want to do is kick back on the couch and veg out.

This is one of those areas where, if you plan correctly, it's not that bad to exercise in the evenings. In fact, you may discover it relieves stress and helps you unwind after a busy day. And it's also a *much* healthier way to relax than alternatives such as heavy drinking or gorging on junk food.

Now, there is a myth that exercising at night keeps you awake. This is simply not true. <u>Check out this link</u> that shows how exercise at any time will encourage better rest, not hinder it.

This article explains how the National Sleep Foundation studied the sleep habits of 1,000 participants and found that an overwhelming majority (83 percent) of people who exercised at any time of day (yep, including late at night) reported sleeping better than those who didn't exercise at all. The results were part of the foundation's 2013 "Sleep in America" poll.

Now that we've covered how exercising in the evening can help you unwind, serve as a stress reliever, AND help you sleep better at night, you really have no excuse not to give it a try.

HOW TO IMPLEMENT

Step One:

Consider joining a gym during the half of the year when it's dark after work, or come up with a plan to work out at home. (In a later section, we'll talk about how to negotiate a gym contract.)

Remember to keep things safe and avoid running or walking outside alone or without reflective gear when it is dark. You can even purchase a headlamp and exercise in parks at night. Like I mentioned before, I always keep a running headlamp in my car for those times of the year when it gets dark early.

Obviously, it might be best to exercise in the dark with a partner and in a relatively safe neighborhood.

Step Two:

Join a gym near your work. Not only will this keep you consistent, you'll also avoid the rush-hour commute that's common in many urban areas. While people are dealing with bumper–to-bumper traffic, you'll be engaged in an invigorating block of exercise. By the time you leave the gym, the traffic will have cleared up.

Step Three:

Be prepared.

Have a workout bag packed with all the items you need for working out in the evening. Pack a small snack to eat in the late afternoon so you don't feel a food craving or a dip in energy. When you are prepared, you are more likely to follow through with exercise.

OBSTACLE (5):

OUTSIDE DISTRACTIONS AND

DISTRUPTIONS

Sometimes, "life" intrudes on a good fitness plan. Okay, who am I kidding? Not sometimes, but nearly *all* of the time.

In adulthood, it's nearly impossible to have plans without them getting disrupted. These distractions often seem relentless, especially the moment you decide to work on self-improvement or establish good exercise habits.

These plan destroyers include:

- Something else to do
- Children who need attention or sick family members
- Inclement weather
- Work problems
- Relationship trouble
- Vacations
- General "stuff happens" situations

Here's the thing…nobody exercises in a vacuum, free from all responsibilities and disruptions.

It's not like the moment you decide to embark on an exercise program, everyone who needs you will suddenly stop needing you. However, if you are smart about how you structure your day and you keep open communication with others, it's not that hard to manage these potential disruptions and *still* be consistent with your fitness habit.

Tactic #21: Communicate with Family

Family members can be your biggest, most unflinching supporters, but they can also make your best intentions to work out seem unattainable.

Common issues include:

- Spouse who doesn't want you to work out
- Kids who need care and supervision (having young kids who need to be watched is especially challenging.)
- Household responsibilities with no one else to pick up the slack

What can you do to solve these very real problems that can serve as roadblocks to exercising on a consistent basis?

Communication is the key.

For example, you can let your spouse know how very important your new goal is to you and request he/she help with the kids for X amount of time at a certain time so you can meet your daily goal. Your daily micro-commitment is not huge, so this really isn't too much to ask.

If your spouse resists, it may be time to sit down and have a heart-to-heart so you can explain why you are working toward these goals. Let your spouse know how achieving the goals can improve your life and the lives of your family members.

Of course, if you are a single parent, this adds another layer of challenge, but it doesn't mean you should give up trying to exercise in the evening if that is the best time for you.

Look for creative solutions. Barter for childcare from a trusted family member or babysitter. Try to get out of work a little earlier so you can squeeze in a workout before picking up the kids. Find a gym that offers daycare facilities (most have them these days), or just plan to do your workout at home after the kids are in bed.

You have options, so don't feel stuck even if you face some challenges or unsupportive family members.

HOW TO IMPLEMENT

Each type of family situation requires its own strategy. Here are a few ideas to help you find creative ways to meet your fitness commitment, even if family members are making it difficult:

Step One:

Buy a treadmill, stationary bike, Pilates equipment, or yoga DVD. Make it a priority to fit exercise in as you can.

Step Two:

Be realistic. With kids around, you probably won't get time for an uninterrupted hour on the treadmill. You may have to get your exercise in bit by bit when you have time. This makes the whole process challenging, but not impossible.

Step Three:

Let your kids know what's going on with you. Once children are past the toddler stage, they can be surprisingly accommodating. Let them know about your desire to stay fit and healthy. If they understand why Mom or Dad is jumping around or running, and they know they will have your attention when you are done, they will help you stick to your goals.

Step Four:

Talk to your kids while you exercise. You do not need a full hour away. Keep the conversation flowing. Let your kids know you love them. Explain to them that just because you need a little exercise "me" time doesn't mean you are not there for them when they need you.

Step Five:

Let them work out "with" you if they desire, but don't force it. You can make a game out of it. Something like Tae Bo is perfect for this because it is exercise disguised as a fun activity.

The best part is that this early introduction to exercise, when you are not "forcing" it, can set up a lifelong good habit for the youngsters. Ultimately, you want to be an inspiration to your kids/grandkids by getting them interested in the joy of exercise.

Step Six:

Communicate with your spouse or significant other (if applicable). Some people feel they are being selfish if they want to exercise because it takes them away from family and work.

These feelings of guilt are more likely to exist if you have a spouse or significant other who doesn't like to exercise and doesn't see the value in it. You can begin to internalize this and start telling yourself that it is morally wrong to make your exercise goals a priority instead of focusing on other people's needs. If this is ringing true for you, then it's time to open up the lines of communication.

Here are some topics to discuss with your spouse or significant other:

- Time has to be reserved for YOU. This is not selfish; it's healthy. We aren't talking about three hours here—you just need enough time to complete a short routine. Clarify this need with your spouse in a kind and respectful way.

- If you have a really hectic family schedule, you can fit in 5 minutes at a minimum here and there. Ask your spouse to support you and encourage you in this mini-goal. When you make such a request, your spouse is likely to come around and support what you are doing.

- Everyone—whether they're a high-powered executive, the President of the United States, or a work-at-home mom— should have some "me time" in their schedule for exercise. Tell your spouse you want to make sure s/he has some "me time" too, and talk about ways you can make sure each of you gets that time.

- Being fit means you will live longer to be there for your family. It also means you will have more energy to get things done. In fact, the more you take care of yourself, the more ability you have to take care of others.

Communication is the key here. The more open and honest you are about your needs, the more you'll discover that people are willing to accommodate your schedule.

Tactic #22: Schedule Your Day to Prevent Interruptions

One major cause of the time crunch that we often feel is how we handle random interruptions.

You know the scenario—you were going to work out, but something popped up that takes time away from it. You have work distractions or the "just one more email" problem. You keep meaning to get started on your micro-commitment, but you have to answer that text, Skype message, email, etc. It never seems to end.

You will always have interruptions. If you let these interruptions dictate your life, you will never, *ever* accomplish anything beyond the <u>immediate priorities</u> of your job and personal life. This is called survival mode—putting out fire after fire as they pop up. This is no way to live, and it certainly isn't a way to thrive and get the most out of life.

In order to break the cycle of interruptions messing up your plans, you have to take back control of your life. You need to schedule your day and set aside certain times for email, Skype, phone calls, and communication with others. **You also need to schedule your exercise appointment**.

I've mentioned this before, but it's worth stating again: *Place your workout appointment at the same priority level as you would a meeting with your boss.*

If you had a meeting scheduled with your boss, you wouldn't blow it off because you had another email come through. No way. You would wait on checking the email until later and get yourself to that meeting.

The same thing is true during your new exercise journey. If you are serious about this thing, you absolutely must make it a priority, or there will always be some little (or big) interruption that *could* get in your way.

There will always be a co-worker who wants to chat or a family member who really needs your opinion, but they can wait until you have completed your micro-commitment to exercise.

You're not asking for a lot of time; they will survive.

Schedule your day and stick to your appointments—all of them—and you will begin to feel more in control of your life and quite proud of yourself for sticking to the exercise habit on a daily basis.

HOW TO IMPLEMENT

Steps One, Two, and Three:

The simplest all-in-one solution to prevent interruptions is to develop the habit of "If-Then Planning."

Start each day by scheduling *when* you'll exercise and identifying every possible thing that could interrupt this activity. Then, make a series of plans for how you'll handle the interruptions if/when they come your way.

Let's take a look at how this will happen:

1. First thing in the morning, identify the time you'll exercise. If it's part of a morning routine, do it immediately.
2. Scan your calendar to see if there is any other obligation that might be a potential interruption.
3. If your workout is outside, check the weather. If it's going to be inclement, then make a plan for an alternative solution (like going to the gym instead).
4. Treat this like an appointment in your life; it's just as important as a meeting or obligation to someone else.
5. Talk to friends/family/co-workers about this time. Make them understand that this time is special to you. The "me time" for exercise is needed to maintain balance, and you will help them once you are done. Ask them not to interrupt unless there is a real emergency.
6. Don't schedule any events or appointments less than one hour before your exercise.
7. Start "shutting down" 15 to 30 minutes before you plan on leaving to exercise.
8. If, for some reason, you get interrupted for the day, use this as an opportunity to create an if-then plan for the

future. Then, if the same problem pops up again, you'll have a strategy for handling it.

Don't underestimate the power of making plans. We often look for subconscious excuses to not exercise, but when you have a contingency plan for every situation, there will never be a reason for missing a workout.

Tactic #23: Pay Attention to Weather

One of the most common and annoying interruptions of them all is the weather. What's funny is that we live in an age of limitless information, yet one of the biggest excuses you hear for people not exercising is they didn't expect the weather to be so wet/snowy/cold/hot/dark. If you're willing to plan a little, weather shouldn't be a factor about 99 percent of the time.

We've already covered a few possible solutions in previous sections, but let's take a look at how to be prepare for any type of weather pattern. All you need is some creativity and a small amount of time, and you'll be ready for anything.

HOW TO IMPLEMENT

Step One:

Start each day by checking the weather. In fact, do this a few days out so you know what's forecasted and you can plan accordingly for the rest of the week. Plan for *when* and *how* you'll exercise given the weather forecast, and pack the appropriate clothing for the exercise and weather you expect.

Step Two:

Consider joining a gym. Depending on the time of year, you can often get a short-term deal on a gym membership that will act as a backup plan if severe weather interrupts your original exercise plan. Rain or shine, hot or cold, you can always go to the gym.

For instance, I'm a member of a gym from December to the end of March. Typically, I'll work out there three to four times a week—when it's too dark, cold, or snowy to be outside. And since this gym is within walking distance of my house, I can get there even if there is a foot of snow on the roads. (This happened twice during this past winter.)

Step Three:

Know how to handle various types of weather.

For example:

Cold weather: Layering is the key to enduring an outside workout on a cold-weather day. Begin with some type of thermal underwear with wicking capability. Layer sweatshirts or heavy shirts over this garment, and end with a heavier jacket, gloves and a hat. With enough layers, you can be nearly as comfortable as you are working out on a cool spring day.

Hot Weather: Light-colored gear with a visor or hat helps beat the heat. Make sure the clothing is loose fitting and has some wicking capability. Stay away from cotton, which absorbs sweat and often leads to blisters, rashes, or chafing.

When it's hot, exercise as early in the day as possible or at the very end of the day. Go to shady places and hydrate often. Don't go as hard as you would on a cooler day.

Mildly Inclement Weather: A little cold…light rain…a little snow…a little wind. Honestly, there's nothing wrong with building some mental toughness in the face of mildly inclement weather.

One mindset that works for me is to *be slightly cocky* about my exercise. If you're willing to exercise when others aren't, you'll feel a sense of validation that you're doing something others aren't doing. Just take it easy on these days, don't push yourself too hard, and always stay safe.

Major Inclement Weather: Snowstorms, nor'easters, hurricanes, torrential downpours, and heat advisories—all of these are VERY dangerous conditions, so do yourself a favor and either skip your workout, exercise in your home, or go to the gym (but skip the driving if road conditions are dangerous). Physical fitness isn't worth putting your life in danger.

Darkness: I consider working out in the dark to be a gray area. While I frequently exercise at night (with my headlamp), it's not something I'd generally recommend to other people. Crime, accidents, and monsters (just kidding) all pose some risks, so it's important to be on guard and aware of any lurking dangers.

If you plan on working out in the dark, it's important to bring a few items:

- Reflective gear, including a vest
- Flashlight or headlamp (if you're walking/running off-road)
- Safety items (like pepper spray) if you're worried about your safety

Like many other strategies in this book, a little bit of planning can have an amazing impact on your exercise habit. Just remember—most mobile phones come with some type of weather app. Simply look at this app on a daily basis and use the information to plan your workouts.

Tactic #24: Handle Major Life Disruptions

A common obstacle that many people have is falling off the wagon after a major life disruption. For instance, one thing I frequently hear is, *"Vacation derails my exercise routine, and I never get back on track."*

If it's not vacation, it could be a number of other things: holidays, the birth of a child, divorce, moving, or a death in the family.

These are major life disruptions, and many people use them as reasons to stop exercising and can't seem to find their way back to their commitment.

The key here is to learn how to face these major life disruptions while keeping your exercise habit intact. Keep in mind that breaking a sweat for 30 minutes will often help you get through these life disruptions, relieve stress, and mentally deal with the challenges you're currently facing.

Of course, there are also times when the disruptions are so significant that you simply cannot keep your commitment to exercise daily. These are the times when it's okay to forgive yourself. The worst thing you could do is pile on the guilt and feel bad because you missed some arbitrary personal goal. Just get through the tough times and get back on plan when you can reasonably do it.

HOW TO IMPLEMENT

Step One:

Be good to yourself. When you can't keep your exercise commitment in the really difficult times, you must forgive yourself. This stuff happens to all of us. We all have moments when life gets in the way of our best-laid plans, so do not beat yourself up. The last thing you need is to feel bad about yourself. Tell yourself you will get started again as soon as you possibly can.

Step Two:

When you re-start an exercise routine, do the bare minimum. It's almost like you're starting over; focus on the small wins and build from there.

As an example, even though I've run 15 marathons, when I have to stop running for a month or so, I start up again with a small goal (for me) of running for 30 minutes. I don't punish myself by starting back with lofty goals. Starting small enables me to get back in the groove of things as easily as possible.

Step Three:

Finally, while you can't often plan for random interruptions, you can plan for travel and events that will happen a few months down the road. Here are a few ideas of how to fit in exercise, even when you're on the road:

(I.) Investigate your vacation destination before you go. Reserve rooms in hotels that have good workout facilities or are located near parks.

(II.) Bring light workout gear when you travel—resistance bands pack well and can be used wherever you are. You may not be doing YOUR preferred sport or exercise, but you can at least make sure you are including regular exercise in your routine.

(III.) Walk around the area as a way to see the sights of the location. Bring a pedometer (like the Fitbit) and try to get in 10,000 steps each day.

(IV.) Check out parks and forestry areas near your travel locations. Why not have a nice walk in the park or enjoy a walking trail while you are visiting a new place? Other fun options to mix things up include kayaking, surfing, and biking.

There is a fine line with disruptions. You should plan ahead and know what you'll do when they pop up. At the same time, keep in mind that you're human and there <u>will</u> be times when you slip. It's equally important to forgive yourself for those occasional lapses.

Tactic #25: Increase Your Energy Levels

We covered this in previous sections, but it's worth going over again. The truth is that it is hard to exercise when you feel a lack of energy.

Remember how we discussed the idea of ego depletion?

This is the phenomenon that occurs when you have utilized so much mental and physical energy throughout the day that you are just too spent to avoid the temptations that come your way in the evening.

Your energy is likely at a low point at the end of the day. The last thing you want to do is work out.

This is the reason so many people drop their exercise commitments when the going gets tough. Don't succumb to the desire to quit when your energy levels are low. Instead, look for ways to increase your energy levels so you can continue to meet your exercise goals.

HOW TO IMPLEMENT

Step One:

Create a solid daily schedule with plenty of healthy habits built in, including proper sleep, good nutrition, and stress management. Having good energy levels throughout the day happens when you regularly make smart choices.

Step Two:

Come up with strategies you can use to increase energy levels, such as:

- Getting a full night's sleep, which we've already covered.
- Focusing on well-balanced nutrition. Consume energy-giving foods—such as bananas, pineapple, watermelon, and healthy grains—close to your exercise time.
- Drinking plenty of water—before, during, and after a workout. If you're dehydrated, you will feel low on energy. Many people who haven't been drinking water are amazed

when they increase their intake because their energy levels go through the roof.

- Consume a *small* amount of caffeine before your workout. Studies show caffeine actually does give you a boost in energy that can benefit your exercise routine. Just beware of the risks of consuming too much caffeine in general. Moderation is key.

- Deal with stress. You can't deny your feelings and emotions when you are stressed out. It's important not to bury them. Instead, deal with them in a healthy way. Call up a friend to chat. Journal about them. Consider seeing a professional counselor. Process your stress as you work out, and you may be surprised how much stress you release as you exercise.

Step Three:

Focus on your exercise commitment—a small amount of exercise to keep your daily habit going. You have to be aware of your patterns and recognize that you're sometimes simply not in the mood to exercise. That is perfectly fine. On these days, don't push yourself to the point of burnout. Instead, just get through your daily micro-commitment. That's enough.

This is exactly why, throughout the book, we emphasize the importance of small wins. If you commit to a small goal, then it's much easier to convince yourself to get started if you only think it'll be for a short time.

Tactic #26: Find a Low-Cost Exercise Program

One major obstacle people often experience is not having enough money to exercise at a nice gym or purchase expensive equipment. The good news is that you don't have to do these things in order to stay in shape.

Exercise doesn't have to cost a thing. You can walk around in any old clothes and get some exercise. Even running can be done in some comfortable clothes and shoes; special running clothes are not essential.

My advice is to spend what you can afford on exercise clothing and equipment, and nothing more. While I do recommend joining a gym to have an alternative solution for when the weather is inclement, you should always be budget-conscious.

When the cost of shoes or exercise equipment makes you balk, compare it to the medical costs people incur because they have neglected their bodies and avoided exercise for a lifetime. Even in the days of Obamacare (or specifically in the days of Obamacare, depending upon your financial situation), healthcare can be really, really, really expensive.

How much better is it to invest in your health and well-being now than to pay for painful and expensive medical care in the years to come?

HOW TO IMPLEMENT

Step One:

Use sites like eBay and Craigslist to search for lightly used equipment or check with family and friends to see if they happen to have stuff in their basement you could borrow or purchase on the cheap.

Step Two:

Focus on exercises that do not require memberships or costly equipment, such as:

- Pilates
- Yoga
- Walking
- Running
- Body-weight exercises
- Apps (like 7 Minute Exercise)

A great exercise program doesn't have to cost money. With a little bit of thought, you can build a routine that can be done everywhere *without* a substantial financial investment.

OBSTACLE (6):
YOU HATE THE GYM

Throughout this book, I've talked about using the gym as a primary (or secondary) place to get exercise. Personally, I have a love-hate relationship with gyms. I've been ripped off by tricky contracts in the past, but I've also used gyms to get through severe, blizzard-like winters. So I completely understand why you might be hesitant about joining a gym.

For many years, gyms have had a reputation of being filled with aggressive salespeople, annoying contracts, limited hours, meat-market dating environments, and guys who "lift things up and put them down."

But if you do your research and choose your gym wisely, you can find a great gym that doesn't cost a lot, is right for your exercise program, and doesn't require you to sign away your firstborn child.

On the other hand, if you're dead-set against joining a gym, then we'll talk about a few alternative solutions.

Here are a few ideas to get started…

Tactic #27: Find the Right Gym

The right gym can completely change your negative perspective on fitness centers. If you know what to look for and how to negotiate the right deal, the gym can become an invaluable part of your exercise routine.

Here are some tips for choosing the right gym:

Consider location. Don't kid yourself into thinking you'll drive all the way across the city to work out at a brand-new gym. If there is one closer to where you live or work, you will be much more likely to go. Other considerations for location include parking (Is it available? Is it affordable?), public transportation (if you need it) and neighborhood safety (in case you want to go at night).

Check out reviews. Use online review sites like Yelp and Google to read user reviews for the gyms you are considering. You can learn a lot about the pros and cons of each gym from these reviews. Also ask around town, or put a question on your social media profile to see if your friends, family and co-workers have suggestions. This insight can be really helpful in making the best selection.

Consider the price. If the price isn't right for your budget, don't sign up. If it's a brand-new gym with all-new equipment and lots of specialty programs and classes, you can pretty much guarantee the price tag is going to be high. It may not be worth the cost to you to have all of these bells and whistles. You may benefit more from finding a basic gym with a fee you can afford.

One more thing…keep in mind that you may be able to negotiate the membership rate, so don't be afraid to discuss the cost with a customer service rep or gym owner to see if they will cut you a deal.

Consider the gym plans available. Before you sign up for a new gym membership, check to see if you are locked into a crazy plan that you'll never be able to get out of in case a medical emergency pops up or you need to move. Ask what their refund policy is and find out if they have a reciprocity agreement with other clubs.

HOW TO IMPLEMENT

Step One:

Conduct a little self-analysis to determine what you *really* need from a gym.

Ask yourself the following:

- When do I like to work out?
- Do I need a gym that stays open late?
- Do I need it for a season (like winter) or throughout the year?
- How much can I spend on a gym?
- Do I want it close to my home or work?
- Do I need additional amenities (like a shake bar, towels, tanning or daycare)?
- What type of exercise program will I follow (weights, cardio or classes)?
- Would I need someone to show me how to do the exercises?
- Do I get a trial day or week? (It's good to use these trial opportunities at the exact time you normally exercise so you know if it gets too crowded at this time.)

Step Two:

Once you are armed with the answers to the above questions, it's time to shop around for the best gym.

Now it's important to remember that it's currently a "buyer's market" for gyms. The gym market has become very competitive. Owners know that most people don't want to be locked into a year-long deal, so don't allow anyone to bully you into a contract that doesn't work. My advice is to simply tell them what you want and say you won't accept anything else.

Here's a list of tips for finding the best gym at the right price:

- **Call first.** Calling makes you less likely to fall prey to high-pressure sales techniques. It's easy to just hang up if you get uncomfortable. It also gives you a chance to shop around. However, don't sign up over the phone. You will want to check out the facilities prior to signing, but calling first gives you a chance to screen your results and decide which gym is worth the visit.

- **Never take the first offer.** Everyone at a gym pays different prices. First quotes are often the <u>most</u> they can get out of you. Be willing to walk away and force the price low enough that they become uncomfortable.

- **Check and double-check the contract.** Just because the salesperson says that is "all the cost" does not mean they really know, or care, if there are hidden costs in the contract. Read the agreement thoroughly and don't be afraid to ask questions.

- **Ask them to waive the membership fee for a year-long contract OR make the contract shorter.** If you are willing to go for a one-year membership, there should <u>never</u> be an up-front membership fee. This is almost always a negotiable variable.

- **Never do more than a one-year contract**. One year is still a long contract, and you do not know what the future holds.

- **Pay in full.** If you have the money and can pay in full up front, you can often get the very best deal possible.

For example, I pay $180 total for three months during the winter. On a per-month basis, it's a lot of money, but I ultimately save money because I know the likelihood of going to the gym the other nine months is small.

Gyms can be great for your exercise routine (or be used to supplement your regular activities). The problem? It's easy to be intimidated by high-pressure sales tactics and an uncomfortable environment. But if you shop around and stick to your guns about what you want, then it's not hard to find the right place for you.

Tactic #28: Build a Home Workout Routine

Working out at home has become a popular alternative to gyms. Between workout DVDs, exercise-based video games, YouTube, and skill-learning websites (like Skillshare and Udemy.com), you can build a fitness routine from the comfort of your home.

The trick is to find a workout routine that works for your space constraints and budget. Both may be limited for you, but this is not a valid excuse to do nothing because there are always inexpensive, and even free, exercise alternatives.

For example, push-ups, sit-ups, jumping jacks and stretching programs—not to mention outdoor activities such as walking or running—require nothing but your time and effort.

Of course, if you have the money to invest, there are *many* expensive options, toys, and tools to make things "easier." Many of them might work as promised, making the fitness program of your choice fractionally easier to manage.

However, when push comes to shove, the biggest and most important variable is YOU and not "stuff" or "space."

Heck, even people in solitary confinement find "space" to exercise in a 6x6 box with nothing but a cot, so there should be no problem finding a place to exercise in your home or backyard.

HOW TO IMPLEMENT

Like I said, there is a variety of home workout programs. Some are a fun way to spend 30 minutes, while others resemble a grueling boot-camp environment. The following are a few resources to help you get started.

Extreme Solutions

If you really want to kick-start your fitness routine with some serious intensity, workout routines like *P90X*, high-intensity interval training (HIIT), and *Insanity* may be what you're looking for.

All three are centered on similar principles: high intensity yields more results. The benefits of high-intensity training include:

- Boosted Metabolism
- Muscle gain
- Increased stamina

P90X is unique from HIIT and *Insanity* because it has a yoga component, which some don't view as high-intensity training (though it is challenging and beneficial).

P90X, HIIT, and *Insanity* are designed to jumpstart your metabolism, challenge your muscles, elevate your heart rate, and truly whip you into shape. While some weights can be used, many of these workouts can be accomplished simply by utilizing your own body weight in a range of plyometric workouts. The amount of power and resistance you get from many dynamic exercises can still be very challenging, even without the use of added weight.

These workouts are best for those who are either looking to take their fitness to the next level or are looking to get back into fitness after a long vacation. These workouts will be a real challenge; however, the results are worth every bit of effort.

Though these workouts are intense and trying, any of the workouts can be scaled. In other words, the moves used in *P90X*, HIIT, and *Insanity* can be altered to match any fitness level.

Fun but Challenging

For home use, workout videos such as those by Jillian Michaels, Tone It Up's Karena & Katrina, and Nintendo can play a helpful role in effectively achieving a higher fitness level from home.

Fitness professional and front woman Jillian Michaels offers an expansive set of workout DVDs.

She essentially has come out with a workout DVD to target all of your fitness needs. *Killer Buns & Thighs*, *Killer Abs*, and *No More*

Trouble Zones all provide you the opportunity to target and tone specific areas of your body.

Get Fit & Fab, Hard Body, Shape-Up, and *Complete Body Workout* all offer a more generalized fitness approach that will improve your fitness levels and strength all the way around.

Jillian also offers videos that act as workout plans: *10-Day Shred & 30-Day Shred.*

If you're truly looking to improve your fitness in all facets, it's helpful to include flexibility and balance exercises in your home workout routine.

This is where a video like Jillian Michael's *Yoga Inferno,* Wii Yoga or Tone it Up's yoga routines can come in handy. Yoga will help you recover more quickly, minimize the risk for injury, and gain a greater range of motion—just to name a few benefits. Yoga also provides a way to improve upon your mind and body connection, reduce stress levels, and create a positive mentality. Optimizing how your mind works is a worthwhile undertaking, as it makes up the foundation of self-belief, motivation, and wellness.

After all, if you do not keep your workout routine fun and energizing, you're likely to abandon it just as quickly as you picked it up.

Fun is an ingredient that is crucial to your workout routine. With regard to home workout routines, the best way to accomplish your goal is to find a video led by a person you feel inspired by. Tone It Up's Katrina Hodgson and Karena Dawn are known for their bubbly, goofy, and motivating personalities that inspire many individuals to get moving and love their bodies.

These ladies have compiled a versatile range of YouTube videos as well as a few DVDs that can help you tone up your body and change your lifestyle for the better. Along with fitness routines, Katrina & Karena offer nutrition plans and advice.

Apps

In a world that is becoming increasingly more technological, fitness routines are no exception to the trend. In scouring the app store on your smartphone, you will quickly notice there is a plethora of apps offering various approaches to fitness.

Fitness apps are unique in the realm of home workout routines because they offer incredible portability and access to workouts anywhere you can get an Internet connection. Many apps don't require any sort of equipment, making them even more practical for the busy, commuting individual. Not only are these apps suitable for home use, but you can take the same routine to your office, workplace, or gym.

The 7-Minute Workout app, for example, is one such app that claims to provide you with an effective, challenging workout using only your own body weight. The 7-Minute Workout app is comprised of 12 high-intensity body-weight exercises (30 seconds per exercise, 10 seconds rest between exercises.) The app itself graphically demonstrates each move, plus it has a countdown timer and instructions through the duration of the workout.

Best of all, this app has a free version, so you're essentially getting a virtual trainer to work with at no charge.

Online Personal Trainer Courses

Udemy is an online resource that allows you to pick a personal trainer, select a program, and implement a fitness routine. On Udemy, you can look at the profiles of thousands of individual personal trainers, learn about their programs, and find out about their experience. You can also read about the logic behind why each trainer recommends a certain type of training.

The benefit of this method is its flexibility. You are able to choose how much you want to spend, who you want to seek advice and training from, and what your goals are. With a personal trainer, you are often able to customize your routine to your body, capabilities, and desires, whereas some videos offer the same exact workout to everyone who uses them. Udemy gives you a lot of choice in the matter, making it ideal for anyone who wants a customized workout routine.

YouTube

YouTube is a fantastic resource for both researching a new workout routine *and* supplementing the exercise you already do. Sometimes, having a visual representation of your workout can keep you inspired, help you practice good form, and motivate you to keep working out; you'll feel like you have a virtual workout partner.

The convenience of YouTube is unparalleled. You can scour millions of workout videos simply by searching key words like "HIIT" or "Yoga" or "Fat Burn." Here are two great channels to get you started:

https://www.youtube.com/user/JillianMichaels
https://www.youtube.com/user/ToneItUpcom

You can find a lot of variety with your home workouts. My advice? Be open to learning new methods, getting out of your comfort zone, and changing up your routine if needed. This will prevent boredom, increase the likelihood of you sticking with a routine, and keep your body challenged.

Remember: A body that is constantly challenged will produce better results.

OBSTACLE (7):
AGE, INJURY AND SORENESS

As we get older, a natural aging process causes our bodies to deteriorate. This is perfectly normal and should be expected. Injuries can build up, and we often can't do what we used to do. However, this doesn't mean we should use normal aging as an excuse not to exercise.

New research is showing that a person can slow the aging process by exercising regularly. Many of the changes attributed to aging are actually caused by a lack of movement.

While no person can stop the clock, slowing the tick is worth the effort, right?

Exercise is not the fountain of youth, but it is a good, long drink of vitality, especially when combined with a healthy lifestyle.

In this section, I'll provide a few simple solutions for getting past the physical stumbling blocks that often get in the way of exercising consistently. By using these solutions, you'll experience a slowing of the aging process and possibly feel better than ever with a little effort.

Tactic #29: Know When You're "Hurt" or "Injured"

There's an old adage when it comes to pain and competitive sports: Ask yourself, *"Are you hurt or injured?"*

People often make mental excuses that they can't exercise because it's painful, but it is important to keep in mind that not all pain is related to an injury. In the next section, we'll talk about what to do when you're injured. But, for now, what can you do about the normal "pain" and discomfort associated with exercise?

Sometimes a good exercise day can cause fatigued muscles, especially if you pushed yourself and "overdid" it. This is natural. Keep at it and the same level of exercise will not cause pain in the future, as your body will become acclimated to the higher level of intensity.

Still, that doesn't stop the pain of fatigued muscles from being de-motivational, does it?

What often develops is something called *delayed onset muscle soreness (DOMS)*, also known as muscle fever, which is the pain and stiffness felt in muscles several hours to several days after strenuous or new exercise.

While this may be normal, it's important to know how to handle the problem of being in pain so you can keep moving forward with building your exercise habit.

HOW TO IMPLEMENT

Here are a few strategies to repair your body when it's sore:

Step One:

Gentle walking. Just sitting still all day is the worst thing you can do for fatigued muscles. Movement stimulates blood flow, which helps muscles heal and breaks down lactic-acid buildup.

Taking a nice, slow walk or walking around for 5 minutes every hour or so may hurt a little bit at first, but this activity will help your muscles heal faster.

Step Two:

Use ice, then heat. Ice has immediate pain- and inflammation-relieving properties. Ice down the area that is in pain; later, apply heat to the sore area to soothe the muscles and prepare them for your next exercise session.

A few helpful bits of information:

- Cold on muscles—speeds healing
- Cold on muscles—helps prevent more damage
- Heat on muscles—*feels* relaxing
- Heat on muscles—short-term pain relief for mild pain
- Cold before heat has long-term benefits. Heat makes it feel a little bit better NOW.

Step Three:

Have a post-workout snack.

Research has shown that consuming protein and carbs after workouts decreases the chances of developing muscle fatigue and pain. Having a small, healthy snack after exercise can truly help you feel more comfortable following a workout. Cherries, specifically, have been shown in studies to be a great after-workout snack that reduces muscle fatigue.

Similarly, there have been quite a few studies showing that consuming protein post-exercise also helps decrease the chance/severity of DOMS from tough workouts.

Step Four:

Find effective pain relief. Here are some examples of medications and pain-relief techniques that might help with your muscle pain:

Ibuprofen: Anti-inflammatory

Acetaminophen (Tylenol): *Not* anti-inflammatory, but does have some pain-relieving qualities

Topical pain relief (Icy Hot, Bengay): Often menthol-based, these creams and gels can soothe painful muscles from the outside in. With this type of remedy, you apply the pain reliever directly to the sore area, eliminating the side effects associated with taking medications.

Caffeine before exercise: While caffeine is not always a good thing, scientific evidence has shown it can be a useful tool in combating those aches and pains when consumed before your workout.

Deep-tissue massage: Scheduling a deep-tissue massage with a professional, licensed massage therapist can be a great reward for completing your daily exercise habit. It will soothe your sore muscles, get out any knots, and help you feel ready to jump back in to exercise the next day.

Omega-3 fatty acids: It is amazing what a simple fish-oil pill can do for you when you take it on a daily basis. Omega-3 fatty acids have been shown to reduce arthritic pain, especially in the neck and back.

In one study it was found that consuming omega-3s in the form of a fish-oil supplement provided pain relief comparable to that experienced from taking Ibuprofen.

You can't let a bit of discomfort hold you back from exercising. If you're smart about how you build up the habit and you do the right things afterward, you should be able to recover quickly. That said, there *will* be times when you get injured, so let's talk about what to do when that happens.

Tactic #30: Consult a Doctor for Injuries

This definitely falls under the "no duh" category, but I'm constantly amazed at how many people will let a simple injury build up into a debilitating lifelong injury that prevents them from ever exercising.

It's always best to consult a doctor when you think you may have an injury. In fact, it is better to err on the side of caution with this.

Whether we are talking about shin splints, chest pains, or painful muscles, it's often difficult for you to know whether it is a normal part of starting a new exercise program or a serious health concern.

How can you tell normal pain from something serious?

The short answer is *you can't!*

When in doubt, see a doctor. If the injury is real, it is better to get treatment right away than to keep exercising.

Sometimes, a person thinks sore muscles are enough of an injury to keep him from working out altogether. This is why it is important to get a full medical check-up before beginning any new exercise routine. You'll get a professional opinion on any actual or perceived injury.

HOW TO IMPLEMENT

Step One:

When you talk to your primary care doctor about an injury, briefly explain your injury and try to get a referral to someone who specializes in sports injuries. It will be to your benefit to schedule an appointment with a doctor in sports medicine. It might seem like extra money to see a specialist, but it's well worth it because this type of doctor has more experience with sports injuries and muscle pain than a primary care physician.

To illustrate this point, for the past eight years, I have had moments where I experience a "clenching" sensation in my chest. Like most people would do, I sought immediate medical attention. My thought was this could be the symptom of an impending heart attack. I even went to the hospital for a week and went through a series of tests to diagnose the problem.

Nobody could figure it out. My primary care physician even made a joke about how running marathons was my own stress test. Since I didn't drop dead, I was *probably* healthy. Real funny, right?

It wasn't until I went to a top-notch cardiologist last year that I got an answer to my question. My pain was caused by something called pericarditis, which is simply an inflammation of the sac that surrounds my heart. It's painful at times, but not life threatening.

The point of telling this story here is, if I hadn't seen a specialist, I would have assumed I had a major heart condition. Perhaps I would have given up on exercising regularly. But when I finally talked to a cardiologist, I received specific, actionable information on how to best handle my situation.

Step Two:

Prepare for your specialist's appointment by having the following in your possession:

- Your personal medical history
- Family medical history
- Detailed descriptions of your symptoms (Be prepared to describe pain as sharp or dull, and give the pain a rating from 1-10.)
- Explanation of how the injury impacts you (If you are a runner, for instance, the doctor should know this, because a sprained ankle impacts your lifestyle.)
- Any questions or concerns you have

One thing to remember…doctors are trained to rapidly diagnose medical conditions. Many times this means they won't spend a lot of time *listening* to what you're saying. So having a list of pre-written questions and descriptions can often help you accurately describe what's going on.

Step Three:

Be sure to ask specific questions if you don't understand what the doctor is saying. You're not stupid if you're unclear about certain term or a piece of advice. It's the doctor's job to make you understand the intricacies and impact of your injury.

Yes, doctors often talk over your head and try to rush you, but this is *your* health, so don't be afraid to ask as many questions as you need to understand what's going on.

To help you prepare, consider this list of important questions to ask, write them down, and take them with you to your appointment:

- *What is my diagnosis?*
- *What tests confirm this diagnosis?*
- *Could this be multiple problems?*
- *Could it be something else?*
- *Do I need surgery?*
- *Will this surgery hurt?*
- *How long is the hospital stay?*
- *Can I expect a full recovery?*
- *Will I need follow-up treatment?*
- *Will I need referrals?*
- *What fitness-related activities do I need to avoid?*
- *How long do I need to stay away from them?*
- *On what schedule can I (gradually) resume my normal routine?*
- *What fitness activities can I do while recovering?*
- *How long can I expect recovery to take?*

When it comes to your health and well-being, it is important to be sure you get the best information and go over all of your options. If a doctor seems unwilling to discuss your concerns or answer questions, find a doctor who will. As always, don't be afraid to get a second opinion.

Tactic #31: Find a Substitute Activity

Sometimes you simply can't do your preferred exercise routine, but this doesn't mean you have a free pass to slack off. The truth is there are numerous exercises that can be done—with so many variations and modifications—that you shouldn't have a problem finding some way to work out.

It's perfectly fine and encouraged to switch up your exercises. Go ahead and get into the habit of experimenting with different activities until you find the ones that work for your fitness level and *don't* aggravate your injury. The point here is to never stop exercising unless you are laid up, unable to do anything at all.

Do some Google searches to find workout plans for peoples with injuries. You will likely find blog posts, videos on YouTube, and even posts from people in your situation who are members of online forums.

HOW TO IMPLEMENT

Step One:

Talk to your doctor and ask for a recommendation on an exercise substitute. This will be your best place to get advice about what to do next. Refer to the previous solution for more information on how to do this.

Step Two:

Find something you can do to help you stay fit when injured. At a minimum, find some kind of movement or activity that acts as a placeholder until you are able to do your normal routine. Keeping this time "occupied" is important, as is keeping your body moving.

Here are some alternative activities to consider when you are dealing with an injury:

- Walk when hurt from running.
- Swimming can be a gentle alternative when muscles are injured. The fluid movement helps to rebuild strength without straining the joints.

- Walk/jog if you normally lift weights and have a shoulder or neck injury.
- Try pool running if you can't do high-impact exercises.
- Ride a recumbent bike if you have a back, neck, or shoulder injury.

Step Three:

Maintain your exercise habit through your injury if approved by your doctor. It's really important to continue setting aside time for your daily exercise.

If you can only do 15 minutes of some stretching or low-impact movement, then that's okay. The important thing is you're staying committed to daily exercise. If you completely give it up while you are healing, it will be that much more difficult to get back into the swing of things when you are fully healed.

Tactic #32: Evolve Your Exercise Program

As we get older, life puts limits on what we can do. Exercise can help us live longer and stay active for a longer period of time. However, as age and injury intrude, your fitness choices narrow.

One of the most significant "habits" you can incorporate in your life is the ability to mentally reframe what you find acceptable for your exercise routine.

Exercises for seniors and those seriously out of shape should focus on simply doing anything that is considered body movement. As you build your habit, do a little more. As your mobility, range of motion, and fitness increase, you can try adding in more challenging workouts. Until you get there, be patient and focus on exercises that are safe and appropriate for your current condition.

HOW TO IMPLEMENT

At the risk of sounding repetitive, the best way to get information is to talk to your doctor. Your doctor is familiar with your medical history and current injury, so find out what he or she recommends. Your medical team knows what is best for you and what you can handle with your current limitations.

WARNING: Before starting any routine or activity, I strongly recommend getting professional, medical approval on the types of exercises that are safe for you to do.

With that said, here are a few exercise habits you should be able to safely introduce to your routine:

(1.) Stretching:

Static stretching (long/slow stretches) helps improve range of motion and mobility.

- Stretch your neck, shoulders, upper arms, upper body, chest, back, ankles, legs, hips, and calves.
- Use slow, deep breaths while stretching.
- Never push to the point of pain.

(2.) Walking:

Use an indoor track, a walking trail, or a safe neighborhood sidewalk.

- Get a friend or family member involved.
- Focus on posture and form.
- Set goals for time, not distance.

(3.) Swimming:

Start slowly and always swim with someone else nearby. This is an excellent, gentle workout.

- Swimming is low impact.
- Water relieves stress on joints.
- Swimming laps in the pool will also help you stretch and lengthen muscles, enhancing mobility.

(4.) Water Aerobics:

Find a local class; it is very popular among elderly people and has many benefits.

- Cardio exercises for those with limited mobility and/or joint issues.
- Strength and endurance with no impact.
- Exercise done in water no deeper than chest height; you do not even need to be able to swim to participate.
- Builds muscle through resistance of movement in water.

(5.) Cycling:

Use a real bike on a trail or a stationary bike.

- Low impact and gentle on joints.
- A recumbent bike at the gym is great for the elderly because it provides more back support than a traditional exercise bike.

(6.) Weight lifting:

Yes, even "older" people can lift weights; it's a great way to build muscle, which is so important to prevent many issues that come with aging.

- Low impact.
- Focus on slow weight lifting, not trying to beat 20-year-old muscle heads. Just do what you can slowly. Repetitions beat out weight per rep.
- Never get to the "pain point." If weightlifting causes pain, either decrease your weight or switch to another exercise.

(7.) Tai Chi:

This is a type of martial art very well known for its defense techniques and health benefits. This martial art has evolved over the years into an effective means of alleviating stress and anxiety. It is considered to be a form of "meditation in motion," which promotes serenity and inner peace.
- Low impact and gentle on joints.
- Improves balance, strength, and flexibility.
- No special clothes necessary.
- Meditative—helps the mind as well as body.
- Focus on breathing helps improve concentration and reduce stress.

(8.) Yoga:

Not only for the bendy and flexible experts, yoga is a wonderful, relaxing exercise for the elderly.

- Use a yoga DVD or class specially designed for elderly people who have a limited range of mobility.
- While DVDs are good for yoga, always take classes first. It is hard to tell how your form is without an instructor.
- Yoga instructors can also walk you through alternate positions and any modifications you need for the poses.

(9.) Gardening:

Gardening is an ideal activity for mind, body, and soul; it encourages productivity and a feeling of accomplishment.

- Gets you outdoors on nice days with some physical activity.
- Gardening stool and some tools can keep you off the ground.
- Has built-in goal and visible results in a nice garden.
- Seasonal—not a year-round fitness goal, but something of a sideline to keep your interest in the milder months.

(10.) Golf:

Is there anything more stereotypically "senior" than golf? But seriously, some stereotypes are built from solid trends.

- Golf is a great workout for those getting older, as it gets you outside and moving for a couple of hours in a pleasant setting.
- Often a social activity as much as a "fitness" activity, which makes it easier and more enjoyable to form a habit.

Even if you're older, there are plenty of opportunities to exercise on a daily basis. Simply talk to your doctor. Then try one of the ten ideas that I just listed. Some might not be for you, but keep trying things until you find something that works for you.

HOW TO BUILD YOUR EXERCISE HABIT

8 Steps for Starting the Exercise Habit

Throughout this book, we've covered a wide variety of obstacles and identified how they hold you back. We also dived into different solutions you can incorporate to move beyond the obstacles you face. We've covered a *lot* of content, so you're probably motivated and ready to get started with your next exercise habit.

That's why, in this section, we'll tie everything together into eight steps that will turn this information into action.

Let's get started…

Step 1: Build One Type of Exercise Habit

Remember back to our conversation of ego depletion, which is "a person's diminished capacity to regulate their thoughts, feelings and actions"?

Ego depletion impacts our ability to form new habits because our supply of willpower is spread out among all the areas of our lives. Because of this, it's important to work on only one habit at a time. That way, your store of willpower can be channeled into completing that one habit, increasing the odds of success.

So what will your one exercise habit be?

Identify it now and learn everything you can about how to do it right. Become an expert in this one exercise or activity.

For me, this exercise has been running. I have lifted weights, swum, done *P90X*, played sports, walked, and participated in many other exercise routines, most of them perfectly fine for getting the job done.

However, the important point is finding something you can do all the time, something that will fit into your life and can be made into a habit that you commit to do on a daily basis, even when you don't feel like it.

Step #2: Commit to the Habit for 30 Days

Some people say it takes 21 days to build a habit, while others claim it takes up to 66 days. The truth is that the length of time really varies from person to person and habit to habit. You'll find that some habits are easy to build while others require more effort. My advice is to commit to a specific exercise habit for the next 30 days (or a month to keep it simple).

During this time, your entire life should be structured around getting *some type of movement* every single day.

Step #3: Anchor Your Exercise to an Established Habit

In essence, the point of this book is the idea that exercise should **not** be based upon motivation, fads, or temporary desire. Rather, it should be instilled in your life to the point it becomes habitual. This often means you do not need fancy exercise routines, just something you can commit to day in and day out…FOREVER.

We've already talked about B.J. Fogg and his "Tiny Habits" concept. What you want to do is to commit to a very small habit change and take baby steps as you build on it. An important aspect of his teaching is to "anchor" the new habit to something you *already* do on a daily basis.

"After I get to my car from work, I will change into my workout clothes and walk for 10 minutes."

"After I wake up, I will turn on my workout app and do my 7-minute morning workout routine."

"After I drop off the kids at the babysitter, I will stop by the gym for my yoga class."

You get the idea. Simply find a habit you already consistently do and then anchor it with a new behavior.

Step #4: Take Baby Steps

We've already talked about the importance of making micro-commitments and focusing on small wins. Think back to our brief discussion of motivation. The danger of relying on motivation alone is that you don't have a backup plan for when you're not in the mood. Really, the only way to make a habit stick is to turn it into automatic behavior. You can do this by taking baby steps and creating a low level of commitment.

The idea here is to create a micro-commitment where it's impossible to fail. It's more important to stay consistent and not miss a day than it is to hit a specific milestone. What you'll find is that when you have a low level of commitment, you'll be more likely to get started.

Examples of zeroing in on a micro-commitment include:

- Walking for just 5 minutes a day.
- Showing up to the gym and doing just ONE exercise.
- Picking ONE app to use to create your daily exercise habit.
- Focusing on stretching and stretching alone.
- Waking up each morning and doing a 15-minute workout, nothing more, for 30 days.

Odds are, these activities seem overly simplistic. That's the idea here! You want to commit to something so easy that it's *impossible* to miss a day. Then, when you get started, you'll often do more than you intended.

Step #5: Plan for Your Obstacles

Every new routine will have obstacles. A large portion of this book is dedicated to working your way through the stumbling blocks that get in the way of your success. When you know in advance what your obstacles are, you can take preventative action to overcome them.

Examples of common obstacles:

1. Time
2. Pain
3. Weather
4. Space
5. Costs
6. Self-consciousness

Prepare and anticipate that these obstacles will come. Then, you won't be blindsided by them. This goes back to the "If-Then Planning" we discussed. Some examples of these powerful "If-Then" statements include:

"If I check the weather and it's raining, then I will work out at the gym instead."

"If one of my children get sick and I can't make it to the gym, I will do my at-home weightlifting routine instead."

"If I have a really bad day at work and don't feel like working out, I will still walk briskly for at least 15 minutes."

Step #6: Create Accountability for Your Exercise

Track your exercise efforts and make public declarations about your new routine. If you remember the Hawthorne effect we discussed, you know you're more likely to follow through with a commitment when you're being observed by others. To stick with this new routine, you should let others know about your efforts and goals.

Post updates on social media accounts, use apps like <u>Chains</u> and <u>Lift</u> to track your progress, work with an accountability partner, or post regular updates to an online community related to the habit. Do whatever it takes to get reinforcement from others in support of your new routine.

Never underestimate the power of social approval. Simply *knowing* you will be held accountable for your habit keeps you focused and consistent.

Step #7: Reward Important Milestones

An exercise routine doesn't have to be boring. Focus on building a reward system into the process so you can take time to celebrate the successful completion of your goals. The reward you pick is up to you, but it's important to celebrate those big moments along the way.

Keep in mind, a reward doesn't have to break the bank. You could check out a new movie, enjoy a night out with your significant other, or simply do something you love.

We tend to underestimate the importance of having "fun" while building habits. Often, though, having a clear reward for regularly completing an action will help you to stick to the new routine.

Step #8: Build a New Identity

Repeating a habit on a daily basis will only get you so far. You can do a lot by committing to a small action, doing it every day, increasing the effort over time and overcoming obstacles. But at some point, you need to go from simply *doing it* every day to making it a part of your core identity. Only then will you stick to it without the constant need for reinforcement.

James Clear often talks about something he calls Identity-Based Habits. The idea here is that you can build a lasting habit by making it a reflection of who you are on the inside. Simply put, you need to believe the habit is part of what makes YOU a unique person.

He emphasizes the fact that most goals (and habits) are centered on a specific outcome (like generating a specific level of income or winning industry-specific accolades).

It's better to decide that the habit is simply part of your identity and then use each "small win" as a way to demonstrate that it's who you are on the inside.

Really, it starts with a shift of mindset.

With a new habit, reinforce this behavior by saying things like: "I'm the type of person who regularly enjoys the ___ type of exercise."

Then, follow through by doing it on a daily basis.

Eventually, your internal identity will match this daily routine.

Final Thoughts...

We've covered a lot of ground in this book, so I hope you are ready to take this information and turn it into daily action.

If the motivation isn't there, you now have a series of strategies to blast past those moments of hesitation.

If your day goes to crap and every obstacle crops up in your path, you know how to exercise—even when you think you don't have the time.

And if you constantly injure yourself, you now know how to prevent these mishaps and engage in alternative exercise programs.

Now it's time for YOU to take the reins and own your personal transformation.

Only you can put one foot in front of the other and take action...*daily* action.

Remember, it doesn't have to be a large commitment.

You are dealing with a micro-commitment—10, 15, or 30 minutes of your time daily.

You can do it.

I believe in you, but more important, you have discovered with this book that you truly do have it within yourself to make this happen.

As you accomplish your micro-commitment day by day by day, you are building a rock-solid foundation for a lifelong exercise habit.

No matter what physical limitations or obstacles are in your future, I know you can get past them.

Enjoy the ride!

P.S. *I would love to hear from you*! While it's *easy* to connect over Facebook, Twitter, or other social media sites, often it's better to have one-on-one conversations with readers like you. So I encourage you to reach out over email and say hi!

Simply write here:

sjscott@developgoodhabits.com

To get started, I would love to hear about the <u>one thing</u> you'll do…this week…to turn this information into action.

Would You Like to Know More?

You can learn a lot more about habit development in my other Kindle books. The best part? I frequently run special promotions where I offer free or discounted books (usually $0.99) on Amazon.

One way to get <u>instant notifications</u> for these deals is to subscribe to my email list. By joining, not only will you receive updates on the latest offer, you'll also get a free copy of the "Bad Habits No More" audio package. Check out the below link to learn more.

Go Here to Get Updates on Free and $0.99 Kindle Books:
<u>www.developgoodhabits.com/free-70hh</u>

Thank You

Before you go, I'd like to say "thank you" for purchasing my guide.

I know you could have picked from dozens of books on habit development, but you took a chance with my system.

So a big thanks for downloading this book and reading all the way to the end.

Now I'd like ask for a *small* favor. **Could you please take a minute or two and leave a review for this book on Amazon?**

This feedback will help me continue to write the kind of books that help you get results. And if you loved it, then please let me know :-)

More Books by S.J. Scott

- *Level Up Your Day: How to Maximize the 6 Essential Areas of Your Daily Routine*
- *The Daily Entrepreneur: 33 Success Habits for Small Business Owners, Freelancers and Aspiring 9-to-5 Escape Artists*
- *Master Evernote: The Unofficial Guide to Organizing Your Life with Evernote (Plus 75 Ideas for Getting Started)*
- *Bad Habits No More: 25 Steps to Break ANY Bad Habit*
- *Habit Stacking: 97 Small Life Changes That Take Five Minutes or Less*
- *To-Do List Makeover: A Simple Guide to Getting the Important Things Done*
- *23 Anti-Procrastination Habits: How to Stop Being Lazy and Get Results in Your Life*
- *S.M.A.R.T. Goals Made Simple: 10 Steps to Master Your Personal and Career Goals*
- *115 Productivity Apps to Maximize Your Time: Apps for iPhone, iPad, Android, Kindle Fire and PC/iOS Desktop Computers*
- *Writing Habit Mastery: How to Write 2,000 Words a Day and Forever Cure Writer's Block*
- *Daily Inbox Zero: 9 Proven Steps to Eliminate Email Overload*
- *Wake Up Successful: How to Increase Your Energy and Achieve Any Goal with a Morning Routine*
- *10,000 Steps Blueprint: The Daily Walking Habit for Healthy Weight Loss and Lifelong Fitness*
- *Resolutions That Stick! How 12 Habits Can Transform Your New Year*

All books can be found at http://www.developgoodhabits.com

About the Author

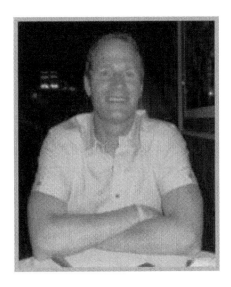

In his books, S.J. Scott provides daily action plans for every area of your life: health, fitness, work and personal relationships. Unlike other personal development guides, his content focuses on taking action. So instead of reading over-hyped strategies that rarely work in the real-world, you'll get information that can be immediately implemented.

Made in the
USA
Monee, IL